Dementia Units in Long-Term Care

Dementia Units in Long-Term Care

Edited by Philip D. Sloane, M.D., M.P.H. and Laura J. Mathew, R.N., M.P.H.

The Johns Hopkins University Press
Baltimore and London

The Johns Hopkins University Press
701 West 40th Street   Baltimore, Maryland 21211-2190
The Johns Hopkins Press Ltd., London

The paper used in this book meets the minimum requirements of American
National Standard for Information Sciences—Permanence of Paper for Printed
Library Materials, ANSI Z39.48-1984.

Library of Congress Cataloging-in-Publication Data
Dementia units in long-term care / edited by Philip D. Sloane and
    Laura J. Mathew.
        p.   cm. — (The Johns Hopkins series in contemporary medicine
    and public health)
    Includes index.
    ISBN 0-8018-4246-8 (alk. paper)
    1. Dementia—Patients—Long term care—United States.   2. Alzheimer's
disease—Long term care—United States.   3. Nursing homes—United
States.   I. Sloane, Philip D.   II. Mathew, Laura J.   III. Series.
    [DNLM: 1. Dementia.   2. Long Term Care—organization &
administration.   3. Nursing Homes—organization & administration.
4. Quality of Health Care.   WM 220 D376385]
RC521.D456   1991
362.1'9683—dc20
DNLM/DLC
for Library of Congress   91-7100

To our mothers

Esther Rendon, who cared for her husband until the day he died of Alzheimer's Disease; and *Grace Heddesheimer,* whose devotion to the nursing profession and to her patients provided inspiration to all who have known her.

Contents

I.   The Challenges of Specialized Nursing Home Care for People with Dementia

II.   Characteristics of Residents with Dementia

Contributors

Kathy Boling, N.H.A., Administrator, Green Hills Center, West
    Liberty, Ohio
Jaikishan R. Desai, M.P.H., Instructor, Department of Economics,
    Davidson College, Davidson, North Carolina
Deborah T. Gold, Ph.D., Assistant Professor, Department of Sociology,
    Duke University, Durham, North Carolina
Lisa P. Gwyther, Assistant Professor, Division of Psychiatric Social
    Work, Department of Psychiatry, Duke University, Durham, North
    Carolina
Lorraine G. Hiatt, Ph.D., Consultant, Environmental Design and
    Aging, New York, New York.
Nancy L. Mace, M.A., consultant in gerontology, Baltimore, Maryland
Laura J. Mathew, R.N., M.P.H., Psychiatry Clinical Nurse Coordinator,
    UNC Hospitals, Chapel Hill, and Clinical Instructor, Department
    of Family Medicine, University of North Carolina, Chapel Hill
Nancy K. Orr-Rainey, M.S.G., Corporate Director, Specialty Programs,
    The Hillhaven Corporation, Tacoma, Washington
Lynn Ritter, M.S.Ed., Therapeutic Recreation Director, Alzheimer
    Special Care Unit, Heartland of Perrysburg, Perrysburg, Ohio

Philip D. Sloane, M.D., M.P.H., Associate Professor, Department of
    Family Medicine, University of North Carolina, Chapel Hill
William G. Weissert, Ph.D., Professor, Department of Health Services
    Management and Policy, School of Public Health; and Research
    Scientist, Institute of Gerontology, University of Michigan, Ann
    Arbor

Foreword

Over the past several years, long-term care in this country has come to include a new component: the specialized dementia unit. In efforts to meet the constantly growing demands for institutionalized care of cognitively impaired persons, both proprietary and nonprofit nursing homes have undertaken the difficult task of designing and implementing dementia units that, at least in theory, attempt to respond to the needs of this special group of people.

The literature has been rife, however, with critical evaluations of some of the units currently in operation. A major criticism has been that many units serve merely as a means of segregating troublesome dementia victims from other residents, without offering the positive and supportive environments that are appropriate and essential to their care.

A major focus of this book is a five-state study comparing the characteristics and outcomes of specialized dementia care units with those of nonsegregated nursing homes. The authors of this carefully controlled study draw a number of optimistic conclusions about dementia units. They believe that the increase in the number of specialized units indicates that the health care system is searching for better ways to care for people with dementia, but they acknowledge that their research presents no clear answers about how to achieve good-quality care. They conclude, however, that the efforts that are being made translate, in many cases, into an improved quality of life. One of the most striking of their findings to support this conclusion is a significant difference in the use of physical restraints, with far fewer persons being restrained in dementia units than in integrated nursing homes.

This book reports the study on dementia units and also deals with topics that are pertinent and fundamental in designing and implementing specialized units. The authors represent a wide diversity of fields and extensive expertise, knowledge, and hands-on experience with regard to dementia care. The book has been written for policy makers in the field of long-term care and for health professionals who are responsible for implementing dementia units and maintaining standards. It also provides guidelines for research design and identifies areas that are in need of careful study to expand our knowledge of ways to improve the quality of life for dementia victims.

Dorothy H. Coons

Associate Professor Emeritus and Associate Research Scientist
The University of Michigan

formerly Director
Alzheimer's Disease Project on Environmental Interventions

Introduction

How best to provide nursing home care for individuals with Alzheimer's disease and related disorders, and what resources are required to do so, are issues often debated by health care providers and policy makers (Brody et al. 1984; Meier and Cassel 1986; Rango 1985; Blazer 1990). While the majority of the afflicted remain at home, more than half of those admitted to nursing homes suffer from a dementing illness.

The Problems of Dementia Care in Nursing Homes

The 1985 National Nursing Home Survey (Hing 1987) reported that 63 percent of all residents were disoriented or memory impaired to such a degree that performance of the basic activities of daily living and mobility were impaired. Other studies suggest that the percentage may be even higher (Sloane and Pickard 1985; Kay and Bergmann 1980; Peppard 1985). These reports imply that a sizable number of cognitively impaired persons live in nursing homes and that nursing home personnel must face a host of issues. Among the care issues unique to this group of nursing home residents are the need for constant supervision because of disorientation, inability to express wants and needs, and a host of disruptive behaviors.

The management of cognitively impaired nursing home residents can be challenging. Studies conducted in nursing homes have described problems in the care of residents with dementia, including: untrained staff, negative or inappropriate staff attitudes toward the residents, little to no treatment offered, frequent use of physical restraints and psychoactive medications to maintain order, an increase in altercations among these residents, and overall deterioration in affected residents' functioning because of low expectations of the staff (Rovner et al. 1986; Teeter et al. 1976; Schmidt et al. 1977; Donat 1986).

The Development of Specialized Units

One response to these problems has been the development of specialized nursing home units termed special care units for Alzheimer's residents. These units, which are referred to as dementia units in this book, represent separate living quarters in the form of a hallway or other closed off portion of the nursing home. They often differ from the rest of the home in terms of physical design and the provision of activities and programming tailored to the needs of residents with dementing illnesses. The dementia unit movement has received public and governmental support, but opinions of health professionals about it are divided. Rabins (1986) and Maas (1988) identified the following advantages of dementia units: specially designed environments, trained and recruited staff, concentrated resources, ability to develop formal behavioral management policies and practices for all residents, alleviation of families' anxiety, and separation of cognitively impaired persons from those who are more intact. Their disadvantages include higher financial costs, difficulty in determining admission criteria, resistance to placement by residents or families, difficulty in recruitment of staff, negative effect of labeling the unit, higher staff turnover rates, and lowered staff expectations. Rabins states that research is needed to determine the effectiveness of these units. He cautions that more experience and knowledge are needed before nursing homes launch a widespread effort to establish dementia units.

Yet the nursing home industry continues to build or renovate facilities in order to open more units. An Office of Technology Assessment report on Alzheimer's disease completed in 1987 stated that, of approximately 22,000 nursing homes in the country, 150 to 200 had dementia units (U.S. Congress, 1987). Based on national survey data collected in that same year, however, Leon et al. (1989) estimated that 7.6 percent of homes nationally had specialized units and that as many as 14 percent will have such units by 1991. Dementia units continue to proliferate even though the question whether to segregate residents in the first place remains unanswered.

Separating nursing home residents with Alzheimer's disease from those who are cognitively intact meets the criticisms: inaccurate diagnosis of dementia may occur, little research indicating that segregation is beneficial, the high proportion and relative heterogeneity of residents with dementia, the right of demented residents to be treated equally, the high costs of operating dementia units, and an expectation that nothing beyond segregation can be done for the demented (Getzlaf 1987; Hall and Buckwalter 1990). Proponents of the traditional, integrated model of care argue that behavioral problems can be managed through a variety of interventions that can be used throughout nursing homes.

Proponents of the integrated model also cite studies indicating that separation may not be helpful. A study conducted in Great Britain on environments for demented elderly persons (Meacher 1972) found that persons in separated environments had fewer visitors and were more likely to want to leave, more likely to be confused, more delusional, and more physically disruptive than the elderly demented who were not segregated.

Another early study (Harris et al. 1977) found that severely impaired persons engaged in little socialization, but when they did so, it was with the unimpaired and not with others like themselves. This would lead one to believe that housing demented residents only with persons of similar cognitive ability would result in little to no stimulation. Cornbleth (1977) found that a special hospital ward for wanderers helped to improve range of motion and physical activity but had no effect on cognitive or psycho-social function.

Adding to the controversy is the heterogeneity of existing dementia units. Ohta and Ohta (1988) examined policy and procedure manuals, reviewed published and unpublished studies on dementia units, made personal observations, and concluded that any research conducted in this area will have to account for the wide differences in care management and philosophy. Perhaps for this reason, few researchers have attempted to measure empirically the effects of dementia units.

What literature exists generally argues in favor of dementia units but is descriptive rather than empirical. Innovative programs, as well as philosophical statements about the units and their potential worth, are common (Peppard 1985; Coons and Weaverdyck 1986; Maas 1988; Hall et al. 1986; Salisbury and Golhner 1983; Novick 1985; Coons 1986; AHCA 1986; Goodman 1986; Johnson 1986; Ackerman 1985; Mace 1989; Millard 1989; Clendaniel and Fleishell 1989). It is now widely recognized that the Alzheimer's resident usually requires a different approach to care from what is offered to other nursing home residents.

There is published information on how to plan a program (Panella 1987; Sanborn 1988; Bleathman 1987), what elements of the structural environment are important (Calkins 1987; Hyde 1989; Roberts and Algase

1988), how to train staff (Mace 1990; Gwyther 1985; Coons 1987), how the unit may result in staff burnout and stress (Wilson and Patterson 1988), how to approach problematic behaviors exhibited in the residents (Rader 1987; Gugel 1988), what recreational and therapeutic activities are helpful in the units (McArthur 1988), as well as how to promote rest and good sleep patterns (Bernick 1988), how to communicate nonverbally when necessary (Hoffman et al. 1988), and how to support family and other caregivers (Roberts and Straw 1987; Hansen et al. 1988). Also among all this information, a basic argument for the establishment of standards of care is made (Koff 1987).

A few studies have attempted to measure effects of the units somewhat empirically. Other research describes a particular approach or conceptual model from which to study empirically nursing home residents with dementia, although it does not specifically discuss dementia units as a treatment (Hall and Buckwalter 1986).

An early study reported on six subjects followed for one to four months without controls. The authors found an improvement in behavioral problems for the six persons (Greene et al. 1985). Three of the six subjects had pre- and postevaluation of mental status. Of these, two showed improvement in cognitive skills, and all three showed affective improvement. Other research reported posttreatment effects such as decreases in wandering, emotional outbursts, and mood disturbances but failed to use control subjects (Hall 1986).

An Australian study found significant positive effects for the family caregivers of residents admitted to a dementia unit. Relief of the burden often experienced by family members was cited as a reason to establish more units, even though there were no measurable effects on the residents themselves (Wells and Jorm 1987).

Benson et al. (1987) evaluated 32 residents of a dementia unit at entry, and at 4- and 12-month intervals. Residents improved in areas of daily functioning and in both mental and emotional status. The best improvement noted was in the area of socialization and personal hygiene.

Cleary et al. (1988) examined the effects of a new dementia unit on 11 residents. The study found that weight loss was curtailed, agitation was diminished, restraint use was reduced, wandering was no longer a concern, and family members were very satisfied. Like the others, this study did not have a control group.

A cross-sectional study conducted by Mathew et al. (1988) showed no measurable differences in functional ability, mental status, or behavioral disturbances in dementia unit residents compared to dementia residents in a traditional setting within the same nursing home, as well as to dementia residents in a traditional setting in another facility. However, some differences were noted in the use of restraints, with dementia units using fewer physical restraints but similar levels of chemical restraints.

However, two more recent studies were unable to provide additional testimony on the value of these units. In their study of four dementia units, Holmes et al. (1990) found "no deleterious or beneficial" effects. The researchers did not, however, control for characteristics of the study population, who tended to have advanced disease and who may have been able to benefit only on a limited basis from specialized care. Similarly, Coleman et al. (1990) found that placement in a dementia unit did not decrease the acute hospitalization rate for these residents. This finding was not expected since the proponents of these units often describe preventive strategies as part of their care.

Thus, the limited number of studies to date leave several questions unanswered. Nevertheless, family members and health care providers must still decide on the course of treatment for Alzheimer's disease victims. Often the choices are few and can offer only palliative relief. Dementia units of nursing homes may now provide new hope. The number and diversity of these programs offer settings in which many questions can begin to be answered.

More data are needed on the outcomes of specialized dementia care to justify costs in time and effort presently going into the units, to justify more widely available governmental assistance, to determine which therapies are effective, to determine which populations can be helped, to help establish standards of care for the industry, and to guide families in their struggle to find appropriate care for the afflicted.

The Goals and Content of This Book

As specialized units emerged, we were intrigued by their potential. Like so many others, we were often faced with the many challenges of caring for people with dementia in the nursing home. We began asking questions from those in the field and conducted a pilot study at a local nursing home with a dementia unit. These experiences led us to propose a detailed study of at least two dozen dementia units. Receiving a three-year grant from the Alzheimer's Association, we embarked on our task of visiting units around the country and learning all we could.

This book presents the results of these studies. In addition, it provides guidelines for new dementia units in separate chapters authored by leaders in the field. Thus, it seeks to integrate research findings with practical recommendations.

We have divided the body of the manuscript into five general topics: overall issues in resident care; resident characteristics; organization and staffing; the physical environment; and activities as therapy. Within the sections we have included, as appropriate, materials from our five-state study of dementia units and chapters by people who are developing innovative programs.

It is our hope that the book will be useful to direct providers of dementia care, administrators of homes, policy makers and those defining standards of care, researchers who continue to probe this area, designers of specialized areas, geriatrics and gerontology specialists, potential funding agencies, and students learning about dementia.

A Five-State Study of Dementia Units: Overview

The study reported in chapters 2, 3, 4, 6, 7, 9, and 10 of this book was conducted between 1987 and 1989. It had the following five objectives: (1) to estimate the number of dementia units currently operating in five states; (2) to describe existing dementia units in terms of auspices, size, age of program, unit goals, admission policies, physical and environmental properties or modifications, staffing, routine treatment programs, range of services, and costs; (3) to determine the characteristics of dementia unit residents in terms of demographics, functional status, activity level, mobility status, diagnoses, behavioral problems, and physical and chemical restraint use, comparing them with a sample of residents from traditional (nonspecialized) units; (4) to determine what is thought to characterize successful units; and (5) to recommend strategies for objectively comparing the effectiveness of the units with that of traditional nursing home settings.

Study methods are presented in detail in the Appendix. In brief, we sampled and studied 31 dementia units (special care units) in five states: California, New York, North Carolina, Ohio, and Texas. These units were selected so that half were in for-profit homes, half in nonprofit homes. We also identified and studied a comparison group of 32 traditional units within nursing homes that did not have dementia units. The nursing homes in which we selected our comparison units were matched to be similar to our dementia unit nursing homes. This method of selecting comparison homes reduces the likelihood that observed differences between specialized and nonspecialized care resulted from differences between the two groups of homes.

Study data from each home were collected during a half-day site visit. During that visit, we gathered data on the home itself, on the unit being studied, and on 10 residents with Alzheimer's disease or a related diagnosis. In comparison homes we studied one unit, defined as an area served by a single nursing station and certified at the same level as the dementia unit with which it was matched. Our sample of 10 residents was selected randomly from all people with dementia diagnoses on the unit being studied.

We collected the following data on all units studied:

- Screening information from a telephone survey
- Facility and unit information from a questionnaire completed by administrative personnel
- Observational information on the physical environment and activities
- Items from the medical record of our sample of 10 current residents and of 5 recently discharged residents with dementia diagnoses
- Data on the function, nursing care needs, and behaviors of our sample of 10 residents recorded by a nursing staff member familiar with the resident, using the Multidimensional Observation Scale for Elderly Subjects (Helmes et al. 1987)
- Observational data on the 10 residents selected for study
- Subjective notes dictated and transcribed after each site visit

To compare our study population with national statistics for nursing home residents, data from the 1985 National Nursing Home Survey (NNHS) were analyzed. NNHS residents with dementia were identified as those whose diagnoses included "senile dementia/chronic and organic brain syndrome."

Our research findings include descriptions of the residents in terms of demographics, diagnoses, functional abilities, and mental status. The environments in which the residents live are described. We also review administrative issues such as admission criteria, bed capacity, and staffing ratios. The actual provision of care is described in terms of planned activities, interaction among those on the units, mobility status of the residents, use of medications, and use of restraints as we observed during our visits. Finances are discussed in terms of revenues and expenditures. In addition, the administrators of the units we visited provided their personal input on common problems they encountered in development of their units. Based on our findings, a typology of dementia care settings is proposed.

Acknowledgments

We are unable to thank everyone who made this project successful but would like to name some specifically. First and foremost are the administrators and staff of the 63 homes we visited, who so graciously welcomed us to their facilities. Our staff and students on campus, including Jaikishan Desai, Margaret Scarborough, Sara Sarasua, Mary Martha

Bledsoe, David Konanc, Sara Marks, Ronna Hill, Roxie Gunter, and Eunice Grossman, worked at different times during the past three years to help with preparing instruments and collecting or preparing data. In large measure, the project was made possible through the generosity of the Alzheimer's Association, to which we are especially appreciative, together with our list of contributors and consultants whose ideas shaped the direction of the book. Additional thanks go to others who advised us on the project at different times, including Carol Hogue, Gail Weinstein, Sue Miller, Debbie Beitler, Catherine Hawes, and Charles Philips.

References

Ackerman, J.O. 1985. Separated, not isolated—As basic as administrative, backing and commitment. *Journal of Long-Term Care Administration*, Fall, 90–94.

American Health Care Association (AHCA). 1986. Journal issue on special care units. *Provider*, May.

Benson, D.M., et al. 1987. Establishment and impact of a dementia unit within the nursing home. *Journal of the American Geriatrics Society* 35:319–23.

Bernick, C. 1988. Sleep disturbances in Alzheimer's disease. *American Journal of Alzheimer's Care and Related Disorders and Research* 3:8–11.

Blazer, D. 1990. What should the federal government do about Alzheimer's disease? *Journal of Gerontology* 45(1):M1–M2.

Bleathman, C. 1987. The practical management of the Alzheimer's patient in the hospital setting. *Journal of Advanced Nursing* 12:531–34.

Brody, E., et al. 1984. Senile dementia: Public policy and adequate institutional care. *American Journal of Public Health* 74:1381–83.

Calkins, M.P. 1987. Designing special care units: A systematic approach. *American Journal of Alzheimer's Care and Related Disorders and Research* 2:16–22.

Cleary, T.A., et al. 1988. A reduced stimulation unit: Effects on patients with Alzheimer's disease and related disorders. *Gerontologist* 28:511–14.

Clendaniel, B. and Fleishell, A. 1989. An Alzheimer day-care center for nursing home patients. *American Journal of Nursing* 7:944–45.

Coleman, E.A., Barbaccia, J.C., and Croughan-Minihane, M.S. 1990. Hospitalization rates in nursing home residents with dementia. A pilot study of the impact of a special care unit. *Journal of the American Geriatrics Society* 38:108–12.

Coons, D., et al. 1986. *A Better Life*. Columbus, Ohio: Source for Nursing Home Literature.

Coons, D.H. 1987. Training staff to work in special Alzheimer's units. *American Journal of Alzheimer's Care and Related Disorders and Research* 2:6–12.

Coons, D.H., and Weaverdyck, S.E. 1986. Wesley Hall:A residential unit for persons with Alzheimer's disease and related disorders. In Taira, E. (ed.), *Therapeutic Interventions for the Person with Dementia*. New York: Haworth Press.

Cornbleth, T. 1977. Effects of a protected hospital ward area on wandering and nonwandering geriatric patients. *Journal of Gerontology* 32:573–77.

Donat, D.C. 1986. Altercations among institutionalized psychogeriatric patients. *Gerontologist* 26:227–28.

Fries, B.E., and Cooney, L.M. 1985. Resource utilization groups. A patient classification system for long-term care. *Medical Care* 23:110–22.

Getzlaf, S.B. 1987. Segregation of the mentally impaired elderly: Debunking the myths. *Journal of Long Term Care Administration,* Winter, 11–14.

Goodman, G. 1986. Confronting Alzheimer's at Newton-Wellesley nursing home. *Nursing Homes,* March/April, 30–34.

Greene, J.A., et al 1985. Specialized management of the Alzheimer's disease patient: Does it make a difference? A preliminary progress report. *Journal of the Tennessee Medical Association* 78:559–63.

Gugel, R.N. 1988. Managing the problematic behaviors of the Alzheimer's victim. *American Journal of Alzheimer's Care and Related Disorders and Research* 3:12–15.

Gwyther, L.P. 1985. *Care of Alzheimer's patients: A manual for nursing home staff.* Washington, D.C.: American Health Care Association and Alzheimer's Association.

Hall, G., et al. 1986. Sheltered freedom—An Alzheimer's unit in an ICF. *Geriatric Nursing* 7:132–37.

Hall, G., and Buckwalter, K.C. 1986. Progressively lowered threshold: A conceptual model for care of adults with Alzheimer's Disease. Paper presented at the annual meeting of the American Association of Neurosciences Nurses, 15 April 1986, Denver, Colorado.

Hall, G.R., and Buckwalter, K.C. 1990. From almshouse to dedicated unit: Care of institutionalized elderly with behavioral problems. *Archives of Psychiatric Nursing* 4(1):3–11.

Hansen, S., Patterson, M., and Wilson, R. 1988. Family involvement on a dementia unit: The resident enrichment and activity program. *Gerontologist* 28:508–10.

Harris, H., Lipman, A., and Slater, R. 1977. Architectural design: The spatial location and interactions of old people. *Gerontology* 23:390–400.

Helmes, E., Csapo, K.G., and Short, J.A. 1987. Standardization and validation of the multidimensional observation scale for elderly subjects. *Journal of Gerontology* 42:395–405.

Hing, E. 1987. *Use of Nursing Homes by the Elderly. Preliminary Data from the National Nursing Home Survey.* National Center for Health Statistics. DHHS publication no. 87-1250. Public Health Service, Hyattsville, Md., May 14.

Hoffman, S., Platt, C., and Barry, K. 1988. Comforting the confused: The importance of nonverbal communication in the care of people with Alzheimer's disease. *American Journal of Alzheimer's Care and Related Disorders and Research* 3:25–30.

Holmes, D., et al. 1990. Impacts associated with special care units in long-term care facilities. *Gerontologist* 30(2):178–83.

Hyde, J. 1989. The physical environment and the care of Alzheimer's patients: An experiential survey of Massachusetts' Alzheimer's units. *American Journal of Alzheimer's Care and Related Disorders and Research* 4:36–44.

Johnson, J.B. 1986. Chris Ridge Village: A service continuum. *Provider,* May, 32–34.

Kay, D.W.K., and Bergmann, K. 1980. Epidemiology of mental disorders among the aged in the community. In Birren, J. E., and Sloane, B. R. (eds.), *Handbook of Mental Health and Aging.* Englewood Cliffs, N.J.: Prentice-Hall.

Koff, T. 1987. Nursing home management of Alzheimer's disease: Establishing standards of care. *Journal of Long-Term Care Administration*, Winter, 15–18.

Leon, J., Potter, D.E.B., and Cunningham, P.J. 1989. Availability of special nursing home programs for Alzheimer's disease patients. Unpublished manuscript. National Center for Health Services Research and Health Care Technology Assessment, Rockville, Md.

Maas, M. 1988. Management of patients with Alzheimer's disease in long-term care facilities. *Nursing Clinics of North America* 23:57–68.

Mace, N. 1989. Special care units for demented patients. *Provider*, May, 10–13.

Mace, N. (ed.). 1990. *Dementia Care: Patient, Family, and Community.* Baltimore: Johns Hopkins University Press.

Mathew, L., et al. 1988. What's different about a special care unit for dementia patients? A comparative study. *American Journal of Alzheimer's Care and Related Disorders and Research* 3:16–23.

McArthur, M.G. 1988. Exercise therapy for the Alzheimer's patient and caregiver. *American Journal of Alzheimer's Care and Related Disorders and Research* 3:36–39.

Meacher, M. 1972. *Taken for a Ride. Special Residential Homes for Confused Old People—A Study of Separation in Social Policy.* London: Longman.

Meier, D.E., and Cassel, M.D. 1986. Nursing home placement and the demented patient. *Annals of Internal Medicine* 104:98–105.

Millard, S.M. 1989. Maintaining control of the Alzheimer's unit. *Nursing Home and Senior Citizen Care* 38(1&2):13–16.

Novick, L.J. 1985. The confused and the lucid: Separation is ultimate solution. *Dimensions in Health Service* 62:23–24.

Ohta, R.J., and Ohta, B.M. 1988. Special units for Alzheimer's disease patients: A critical look. *Gerontologist* 28:803–8.

Panella, J. 1987. *Day Care Programs for Alzheimer's Disease and Related Disorders.* New York: Demos Publications.

Peppard, N.R. 1985. Alzheimer special-care nursing home units. *Nursing Homes* 34:25–28.

Rabins, P.V. 1986. Establishing Alzheimer's disease units in nursing homes: Pros and cons. *Hospital and Community Psychiatry* 37:120-21.

Rader, J. 1987. A comprehensive staff approach to problem wandering. *Gerontologist* 27:756–60.

Rango, N. 1985. The nursing home resident with dementia: Clinical care, ethics, and policy implications. *Annals of Internal Medicine* 102:835–41.

Roberts, B., and Algase, D. 1988. Victims of Alzheimer's disease and the environment. *Nursing Clinics of North America* 23:83–93.

Roberts, J., and Straw, L. 1987. Taking care of caregivers. *American Journal of Alzheimer's Care and Related Disorders and Research* 2:26–32.

Rovner, B.W., et al. 1986. Prevalence of mental illness in a community nursing home. *American Journal of Psychiatry* 143:1446–49.

Salisbury, S., and Golhner, P. 1983. Separation of the confused or integration with the lucid? *Geriatric Nursing* 4:231–33.

Sanborn, B. 1988. Dementia day care: A prototype for autonomy in long-term care. *American Journal of Alzheimer's Care and Related Disorders and Research* 3:23–33.

Schmidt, L.J., et al. 1977. The mentally ill in nursing homes. *Archives of General Psychiatry* 34:687–91.

Sloane, P., and Pickard, G. 1985. Custodial nursing home care: Setting realistic goals. *Journal of the American Geriatrics Society* 33:864–67.

Teeter, R.B., et al. 1976. Psychiatric disturbances of aged patients in skilled nursing homes. *American Journal of Psychiatry* 133:1430–34.

U.S. Congress. Office of Technology Assessment. 1987. Losing a million minds: Confronting the tragedy of Alzheimer's disease and other dementias, OTA-BA-323. Washington, D.C.: Government Printing Office.

Wells, Y., and Jorm, A.F. 1987. Evaluation of a special nursing home unit for dementia sufferers: A randomized controlled comparison with community care. *Australian and New Zealand Journal of Psychiatry* 21:524–31.

Wilson, R.W., and Patterson, M.A. 1988. Perceptions of stress among nursing personnel on dementia units. *American Journal of Alzheimer's Care and Related Disorders and Research* 3:34–39.

I

The Challenges of Specialized Nursing Home Care for People with Dementia

1

Defining Quality of Care for Nursing Home Residents with Dementia

KATHY BOLING AND LISA P. GWYTHER

There have been a number of attempts to define the quality of care for residents of nursing homes. The government does it through regulations, and most long-term care organizations do it by setting their own standards of quality assurance. In this chapter we will go beyond these measures to identify a special philosophy of care and to describe how it relates to the most practical aspect of life for persons with dementia.

The Philosophy of Specialized Dementia Care

Care denotes what is done by others to and for the resident. In evaluating nursing homes, we believe that we should include more than care and that a more inclusive term should be used: the quality of *life*. This concept is much more adequate for establishing a philosophy and standards for the nursing home in relation to all residents, but especially to persons with dementia. Certainly excellence of care and the manner in which it is given have much to do with the quality of a resident's life. But the quality of life is affected by the total environment, including all relationships the resident experiences.

Every person, including every resident of a nursing home, has the basic right to thrive, to flourish, to be treated with dignity, and to function at the highest level possible. If we believe that each person is unique, the preceding statement expresses a philosophy that would lead us to recognize that all care and, to the extent possible, the setting in which it is given, should be special to the individual. In an institution, of course, there are limits within which persons must live. But creative caring and concern for the quality of each resident's life must inevitably result in some special approaches to persons with dementia.

High-quality care extends beyond the nursing home's concern for residents. It includes concern for the emotional well-being of family members or significant others. The quality of their life will have been greatly affected by the circumstances that led to admission of the resident to the nursing home.

Many of the issues we will discuss relating to the quality of life for persons with dementia are generic to all settings. But some issues—for example, physical design as part of the environment—imply a specialized setting for such persons in a nursing home. Because the pros and cons of integrated versus segregated settings are a general theme of this entire book, not all of the issues involved are raised here. But it is important to relate the concept of the quality of life (versus simply the quality of care) to the question of segregation of persons with dementia such as Alzheimer's. Adequate care using special approaches can be given by well-trained staff, sufficient in number, to persons with dementia who are integrated with other nursing home residents. It is the belief of many, however, that the specialized dementia unit can offer greater opportunities to support a high quality of life—dignity, optimal functioning, and the right to flourish.

Perhaps an illustration will make the point.

Mary has Alzheimer's disease and lives on a unit of 30 persons who have a variety of chronic disabilities. The chronic conditions are mostly physical rather than cognitive. The staff on this unit have been trained in caring for persons with dementia, and the ratio of staff to residents is somewhat higher than required by regulation. The staff has tried to educate other residents on the unit about the unique problems suffered by persons with dementia. Mary frequently leaves her room and seems to look for something or someone. She wanders down the hall into other rooms, picking up items or rearranging things. One day she wanders into Ethel's room, and Ethel is intolerant of the intrusion. She shouts, "Get out of my room! Someone get this crazy woman out of my room!" A nursing assistant hurries in just as Mary is about to throw a vase at Ethel. She calms Mary, distracts her, and leads her back to her room. Mary is soon up wandering again, but she is guided to the morning's group activity, a painting class. Mary's attention span is short, however, and she soon disrupts the activity for other residents, who communicate their frustration. Later in the day, Mary appears in the hall with a slip over her dress and hose over her shoes, just as her daughter comes to visit.

In the above encounters, what happens to Mary's self-esteem? What about her dignity? What about her daughter's feelings about her mother and about the home? What kind of emotional environment exists for Mary in these group activities and in general? Will she not continue to "look for something or someone"? It is our contention that the quality of Mary's life could be significantly enhanced in a separate unit whose entire philosophy, design, and programming is directed toward the needs of persons with dementia.

Simply segregating people or groups by diagnosis, function, or ability to pay, however, without a significant individualization of care plans, can lead to nothing more than "warehousing." It may relieve the cognitively intact residents from the stresses of dealing with persons with dementia, but it denies the impaired residents the right to flourish.

What, then, are the principles of specialized care and life for dementia residents? In the following pages, we will present and discuss 10 principles reflecting a philosophy that supports a high quality of life for demented residents like Mary.

The Principles of Specialized Dementia Care

The principles of a high quality of life set forth here are not necessarily exclusive to dementia sufferers. It is in the practical application of these principles that differences become apparent. Cognitively impaired persons require some unique environmental characteristics and care approaches.

Ten basic principles of a high quality of life for these people are listed in table 1.1. Each is briefly discussed below.

1. There is a clear commitment on the part of the organization to provide specialized (appropriate) care and services. This commitment is seen not only in a stated purpose but in allocation of resources (both human and financial), admission and discharge criteria, and the flexibility to respond to changing needs and to new knowledge gained through research or experience.

2. A trained staff integrates the skills of all relevant disciplines. The staff members communicate with each other and are flexible enough to take on nontraditional roles as needed.

TABLE 1.1   The Principles of Good-Quality Dementia Care

Organizational commitment

Trained interdisciplinary staff

Accommodation of resident's preferences

Preservation of dignity

Identification and treatment of excess disability

Family involvement

A balance between safety and freedom

Ongoing assessment and care planning

Recognition and support of staff

Innovation

---

3. Individual resident preferences and customary routines are accommodated. Residents are not pressed into a schedule or expected to perform in a certain manner in order to be accepted. Therapeutic approaches are fully individualized.

4. Dignity is preserved. The resident is protected from negative or embarrassing feedback or criticism and is treated as fully adult. This principle is manifested in many ways, from facility design to tone of voice used by staff to types of activity promoted.

5. Excess disability caused by factors other than the dementia, such as visual impairment or overmedication, is identified and treated, spared functions are preserved or enhanced, and lost abilities are compensated for.

6. Family members or significant others are involved in planning and providing care to the extent they are comfortable. They are also the recipients of support, information, and education by the staff. As a result, families have realistic, informed expectations about the course of the dementia and the care that may be given.

7. The environment is safe, allowing the resident some physical freedom and a sense of security. Such a setting permits positive emotions of pleasure, comfort, and belonging to be experienced by the person with dementia. This is important for one who appears to have lost most of the past, knows no future, and lives moment by moment.

8. There is ongoing assessment of each resident and response to changing needs.

9. Staff needs are recognized and supported.

10. Problem solving through experiment and innovation is supported. Where possible and appropriate, there is interest and participation in research.

Guidelines or principles are of little value unless translated and applied. Consequently, in the following section, we address the application of these principles. In our discussion, the reader should learn how these principles relate to the quality of life in every aspect of its meaning.

The Application of the Principles

All the philosophies, principles, and goals we can develop mean nothing to persons with dementia until we allocate the necessary resources and move into action. In the pages that follow we discuss the aspects of nursing home organization and of day-to-day care that support a high quality of life for unit residents. Scenarios and real-life examples are used to reinforce major points.

THE PHYSICAL ENVIRONMENT AND DESIGN

An overall goal is a safe, prosthetic, and enriching physical environment that accommodates changing needs. A well-designed, segregated area or special dementia unit, coupled with a truly individualized therapeutic approach by well-trained staff, has fewer restrictions, makes up for cognitive and functional deficits, and provides targeted, meaningful enrichment for persons with dementia. Furthermore, such an environment lessens staff stress.

The Physical Environmental Characteristics of an Ideal Unit

As is discussed in chapters 10 and 11, dedicated environments have many design options. Whatever the physical layout and interior design, our philosophy calls for certain characteristics.

The design creates comfortable, secure, and identity-enhancing surroundings. Currently, such design choices have to be based on the experience and shared wisdom of long-term care professionals, since research on what is "therapeutic" provides few definitive guidelines. Each facility should consciously evaluate its own effectiveness and use these findings to improve the quality of its care.

It seems important to consider the regional, cultural, and ethnic background of residents before defining what is comfortable. For example, a unit serving a rural area in the Midwest, where residents have led relatively quiet farm or small-town lives, is small, homey in a country style, with controlled stimulation. A facility located in the Southwest, with residents of Mexican descent who lived in large families in colorful surroundings, has a successful larger unit with many colorful decorations, music, dancing, and more noisy activities. The residents obviously are comfortable with this. They would probably be uneasy and more apathetic in a more neutral setting.

The space in a high-quality unit is appropriate to the functional levels of its residents. If we can say anything definitive about Alzheimer's, it is that its effects are highly variable. Space as well as programming must reflect this heterogeneity and allow for changing needs over time. Ideally, appropriate (and often different) environments should exist within a nursing home for persons in the early, middle, and later stages of dementia. The choice between segregation and integration with cognitively unimpaired persons comprises design and program options.

The ideal environment provides cues that use all the senses. The possibilities here, both for success and failure, are almost limitless. Examples of cuing include the use of signs with words or symbols (such as a stop sign on a door not to be opened or a symbol of a toilet or the word "bathroom" on the bathroom door), door handles covered with a rough material to discourage use, pictures or objects relating to the residents' earlier lives located at room entrances, and things to touch. Some facilities have experimented with "interactive art" with mixed success. Such artwork usually consists of multitextured, three-dimensional objects that residents are encouraged to touch.

High-quality physical design balances the resident's safety and the right to personal freedom. A well-designed unit allows room for moving about without interfering excessively with others' lives. Private rooms also encourage this. The space is limited enough not to cause exhaustion from uninterrupted walking. Access to outdoor areas is important for many persons, and these areas can be secured by attractive fencing or natural hedges. Ideally, a unit should be designed so that locked doors are unnecessary. Amenities such as a raised garden, porch swing, simple adult games, and a comfortably furnished patio promote a natural, homey lifestyle and can be used to support therapeutic programming.

A warm, intimate social atmosphere should be created. This suggests small units accommodating a family-size group. In larger units, a small "neighborhood" area may create such an atmosphere. Several successful units are designed for 8 to 10 persons, with private rooms opening directly into the main living area. Thus, when persons leave their rooms there is no need to find another place to go. They are immediately with a few other persons who, facilitated by the staff person, represent "family."

The high-quality unit is designed with inviting public areas, places for small groups, and access to privacy. It is important for families, and especially spouses, to feel that they have options for either privacy or public socializing when visiting their relatives.

A unit that is designed on a social (residential) rather than a hospital model allows the staff to observe without intruding upon the residents. An unobtrusive staff desk as part of the common area furnishings is often ideal. This allows a staff person to interact, observe, and be "one of the

TABLE 1.2 Selected Measures of the Quality of Care for Nursing Home Residents with Dementia

---

Process of care
    Amount and quality of social interactions
    Emotional quality of unit
    Chemical restraint use
    Physical restraint use
Resident function
    Alertness and activity levels during day
    Level of function relative to potential
    Rates of disruptive behaviors
    Physical activity and muscle tone
    Maintenance of ideal body weight
    Incidence of constipation and skin breakdown
    Resident's sense of being at home
Staff function
    Employees from other nursing home areas volunteer to work
        on the unit
    Rates of absenteeism and turnover
    Morale
    Stress levels
    Sense of teamwork
Family satisfaction and involvement
    Satisfaction
    Visitation and participation rates

---

family" while carrying out necessary functions. Of course, well-placed locks and storage areas are needed to protect records, medications, and anything harmful to residents.

Key Outcomes

If our ideal unit has the physical characteristics discussed above, it will contribute to desirable outcomes. Table 1.2 lists selected outcome measures that can be used to evaluate dementia units. In the section below, we discuss the ideal dementia unit, highlighting those outcomes that should be particularly influenced by the physical environment.

The need for chemical and physical restraints is minimized. Alternatives to both types of restraint are effective in many situations. A physical restraint may occasionally be needed for a person who is not ambulatory and cannot remember that fact, to prevent severe injury from getting up without assistance. Pharmacological restraints are occasionally needed to control severe behavioral problems. Supported by a well-designed environment, however, minimal restraint use can be achieved.

Disruptive behavior is reduced. Note that we do not say it is eliminated. For some residents the best techniques of design and therapeutic approach cannot totally eliminate disruptive behavior. But the special unit can at least reduce its effect on others and the resident herself. A case in point is "Emma," who has the unique ability to smile and hug one minute and, with no external provocation whatsoever, turn instantly with a slap or a punch and a string of profanity. Emma is a delight in her happy moments and a real challenge at the other times because other residents are afraid of her and, of course, are not safe. However, the design of the unit where Emma lives, with the doors of private rooms opening directly into the common area, allows her to move about safely, converse, observe, and be included in the group while remaining in her room separated by a Dutch door. Yes, this is a form of restraint (which is the state's rationale for allowing the Dutch door), but it is safe and humane, and Emma responds well to it.

The emotional quality of the unit is positive. How is "emotional quality" defined and measured? Such things as emotional outbursts, catastrophic reactions, incidents of positive words or touches, and even facial expressions can be quantified. Informal observation can also provide useful information. In the ideal unit, overall calm prevails most of the time, and interactions are positive both between staff and residents and among the residents themselves.

Residents are also satisfied with their freedom of movement. The design of the unit contributes to this emotional quality overall by reducing confusion, enhancing way-finding, promoting independence and security, and removing extraneous stimulation.

The residents are in better physical health because they can be safe and active at the same time. Physical activity produces better muscle tone, appetite, weight, and elimination. These effects are measurable but difficult to document without controls or changes in an environment, both of which may be undesirable from an ethical perspective. However, such changes are often observed in persons who move from a traditional nursing home setting to a special dementia unit. It should be noted, however, that even the best unit cannot prevent the deterioration that comes with progression of the disease.

Residents are comfortable and have a sense of belonging, of being at home. It is not unusual for a dementia unit resident to tell family or staff who have taken her out of the unit, "I want to go home now." It is clear that a more intimate environment meets the special needs of persons with dementia, producing comfort and a sense of "being there" after their homes of the past have been forgotten.

SPECIALIZED STAFF

The selection and training of the staff for special dementia care is probably the most important element in creating the best quality of life for the residents. It is, after all, the human element that is most important; no amount of programming or building design can compensate for inappropriately prepared or recruited staff. (This is, of course, true for other areas of the nursing home as well and, indeed, for any human services).

Selection

It is vitally important that staff assigned to care of persons with dementia, whether on or off a special unit, be chosen on the basis of their values, motivation, and personal qualities, rather than simply availability, seniority, or even completion of special training. Some values and qualities that are desirable for persons working in the dementia setting are:

- *Open-mindedness.* A willingness and ability to learn new facts and try new techniques are essential.
- *Respect.* A demonstrated attitude of respect for the dignity of impaired persons must be present. Ideally, it will have been demonstrated through previous work within the nursing home.
- *Flexibility.* A special unit often requires a change of pace, of schedules, and approaches.
- *Creativity.* The unique challenges of caring for persons with dementia require sometimes unorthodox, intuitive, creative approaches to programming and to problem solving.
- *Patience.* It requires patience to match a resident's pace, to repeatedly try other approaches to accomplish a task, and to tolerate confusion and the repetition of the same themes, questions, and behaviors.
- *Energy.* Staff must be willing to expend energy to establish and guide relationships and to lend energy to apathetic or withdrawn residents.
- *Sensitivity.* Positive nonverbal skills and sensitivity to the feelings of others should be present.
- *Warmth.* Staff should be able to communicate caring through kind words, smiles, hugs, handholding, and other expressions of warmth.
- *Sense of humor.* All staff who work with dementia residents need the ability to find and express joy, especially through humor and a capacity to laugh at oneself.
- *Self-awareness.* A relatively high degree of self-awareness is important, especially when dealing with irrational interactions. The staff person must know her limits and weaknesses.

A staff member who is very task or efficiency oriented, works at a fast pace, or depends on positive feedback from residents for motivation is unlikely to be very comfortable in a direct care situation with an exclusively dementia group.

A diverse staff is an asset. Some impaired residents respond intuitively and quite positively to staff who remind them of someone. Staff members of different races, ages, sizes, genders, and cultures may all become special to specific residents.

It is ideal to have staff members volunteer to work with dementia residents, but some need encouragement or a challenge to try something new. Anyone considering such a position should observe and talk to those already working on the unit. Some staff respond to the opportunity to do something first, to be part of a demonstration that will receive considerable attention.

The key to an excellent staff is to recruit members with the positive qualities outlined above, then further develop these qualities through training. Finally, staff should be encouraged to develop autonomy and to participate in care planning.

Training

Beyond the training for their jobs in nursing, activities, social service, housekeeping, or maintenance, staff members who are involved in any way with special dementia care need specialized training. It is generally agreed that when staff understand *why* something should be done, they do a better job.

This specific training cannot be done in a couple of hours with a few videos. The minimum of three hours required by the federal government as part of the recently mandated 75-hour training course does not adequately prepare a nursing assistant to work effectively with demented nursing home residents. Chapter 8 discusses staff training and provides curriculum guidelines for nursing staff.

It is ideal to develop separate formal classes for nurses, nursing assistants, and other staff, with some overlap. Also, at least nurses and nursing assistants need regular refresher courses and in-service training.

Staffing Characteristics of the Ideal Dementia Unit

All staff members, even the maintenance personnel, have an understanding of dementia. They have received training in dementia care, including how best to interact with residents. Nonverbal as well as verbal approaches are used that communicate acceptance and ease—something that demented persons seem to understand and appreciate well into advanced disease.

Staff roles are flexible. Traditional roles and boundaries of nurses, nursing assistants, housekeepers, and activity personnel are blurred or modified in order to unify and enhance the residents' interpersonal environment. For example, the activity staff may enable the nursing assistants to do a variety of activities by giving them ideas and providing materials. This reduces the number of different persons entering the resident's home, provides consistency, and contributes to a calm but enriched atmosphere.

An example supports the need for staff flexibility.

> For some unknown reason, Doris (a resident) thinks that a certain housekeeper is her daughter. Whenever the housekeeper is in the unit, Doris is at her side, chatting and "helping" her. As a member of the therapeutic team, the housekeeper provides Doris with familiar activities (dusting, dumping wastebaskets, running the vacuum), then sincerely praises and thanks her for the job she has done. Doris's self-esteem is enhanced and her energies find an appropriate outlet. The housekeeper contributes to the stability of one person and, therefore, of the group, rather than simply being another staff member moving about the unit. Doris needs to be "special." Having a special relationship with the housekeeper contributes to her quality of life.

Staffing patterns are consistent, yet flexible enough to accommodate the changing needs of residents. Consistency of staff allows relationships to develop and reduces residents' confusion. There are sufficient trained staff to cover for breaks, illnesses, and emergencies. Trained backup staff are available if extra help is needed; temporary staff from agencies or nursing pools, which can impair quality, do not need to be brought in.

Ideally, when a resident needs temporary additional care, as during a short-term illness or following a broken hip, she is not moved off the unit. Instead, extra staff are temporarily moved to provide the additional care.

The staff receive support, respect, and recognition from supervisors. This may come in many forms. Some examples are providing access to professionals in mental health and providing opportunities for interaction and communication away from the work setting. One facility "buys" a monthly case consultation conference with university health professionals for staff members at all levels. During that conference, any staff person may bring up a unit resident for discussion, brainstorming, and recommendation. Pizza or other refreshments may accompany occasional sessions for problem solving on one issue, or to provide mutual support for dealing with a death or a difficult situation. One facility periodically gives a group of nursing assistants $20 to $30 to shop for activity supplies together, and $5 each for lunch on the shopping trip.

Finally, regular care conferences provide opportunities for all staff members to have input into residents' care and decision making.

Key Outcomes

Some positive yet realistic outcomes of proper selection, training, and support of a multidisciplinary staff are listed below (see table 1.2):

- Employees volunteer to be special dementia care staff.
- Absenteeism and staff turnover are reduced.
- Staff stress is managed, burnout is rare, and good morale is maintained despite the incurable nature of the disease afflicting the residents.
- The staff have realistic expectations of resident function and demonstrate a working knowledge of therapeutic programming, behavior management, and approaches to families.
- Teamwork is apparent through cooperation and the flexibility of professional boundaries.

THE THERAPEUTIC PROGRAM

The overall goal for a dementia unit is similar to that for any residential therapeutic program: to enhance function and maintain optimum quality of life within the limits or constraints of disability.

To achieve this goal, a program must include identification and treatment of excess disability. It must support and enhance spared function. It must compensate for lost abilities through environmental and social strategies. In addition, an effective approach includes searching for underlying causes of behavior disturbances and alleviating them if possible. Examples include pain that cannot be expressed verbally, constipation, or certain sights or sounds that relate to an unpleasant past experience.

Care must be based on resident need or preference, rather than the convenience of the staff or organization. This requires thought and flexibility. It means that staff must frequently forego the planned resident schedules for meals, arising, going to sleep, bathing, or planned activities.

Assessment

An intake interview and assessment before admission helps to prepare both the family and staff for a smooth transition of care with few surprises. It must be unhurried and should include a medical, personal, and family psychosocial history, as well as functional and mental testing. Further assessment takes place after admission and becomes an ongoing process. Details on resident assessment are provided in chapters 5, 12, and 13.

A consistent evaluation process can monitor mental status, functional capabilities, and activities of daily living over time. Assessment should be repeated at appropriate intervals as part of ongoing case planning and monitoring. This allows the staff to base care and activities on a realistic appraisal of the resident's abilities, neither expecting too much and causing the resident to experience failure, nor expecting too little and causing unnecessary dependence or helplessness.

The Process of Care in an Ideal Unit

A program of caring goes beyond the standard assessment and routine care plan. It addresses issues of the quality of life for both the resident and the family.

There is multidisciplinary care planning for each resident and consistency in carrying out the plan. The care plan is based on carefully gathered assessment data. The initial planning includes professionals representing medicine, nursing, rehabilitation, social services, dietary, and activities. Family should also be represented. Periodic conferences discuss each resident and include the family, nursing assistants, and housekeepers, as well as professionals.

The care plan addresses not only symptomatic behavior but seeks to anticipate and prevent potential problems. Behavior is managed by identifying and treating the underlying causes and preventing exposure to potential precipitating events.

The caring program includes a specified role for family members, if they are available. Family members' roles should be comfortable for them, not just convenient for staff. For instance, a daughter may find it difficult and uncomfortable to feed her mother but may welcome the opportunity to groom her mother's nails during a visit.

Feelings and needs of family members are also addressed by the program, as in the case of Fred's wife, who had cared for him as long as she could before placing him in a dementia unit. She told the staff she was lonely, and that the hardest times were meal times alone. The staff suggested she plan her visits to coincide with his meal and eat with him. Staff arranged for the couple to have a small table to themselves. The staff also supported her need for intimacy and respected the closed room door when she wanted privacy.

Activities in the ideal program always support goals that are appropriate, meaningful, and individualized. They allow success and pleasure and reinforce capabilities. These goal-oriented activities may range from sensory stimulation to physical exercise, to cognitive and intellectual pursuits. Many activities are designed to create social opportunities. For example, sitting in a large circle and bouncing a large light ball from person to person is a simple interactive activity that can stimulate socializing while it provides physical exercise. Further details about goal-based activities are provided in chapters 12 and 13.

In planning activities, it is important to remember that a person with dementia lives very much in the moment. Creating momentary pleasure is a worthy goal. A person with dementia does not remember an activity an hour later but may retain the pleasure. A pretty autumn day may create images of pleasures long past. A hug of acceptance may not be remembered, but it sets the tone for the next few hours.

Above all, high-quality activities for persons with dementia are on an adult level, no matter how simple. Successful activities often use skills learned long ago, such as washing dishes, folding clothes, shelling peas, or sanding wood.

Another characteristic of special caring is flexibility. "Going with the flow" of the residents is far more important than bedmaking, having everyone dressed by 9:00 A.M., doing an activity at 10:00, or making sure John has his bath on Thursday evening. Being creative with new approaches is another aspect of flexibility. For example, John does not want a bath. The staff person will not push or insist. Instead, she returns in a few minutes using visual stimuli: a wet washcloth, soap, and towel. John still says no. A half hour later she brings John his bathrobe and body powder. John has relaxed and goes along for the bath.

One area where flexibility is important and easily accommodated in a special unit relates to eating. Eating often becomes in increasing problem in progressive dementia. If there is resistance to sitting at the table, a tray may be placed wherever the resident is willing to sit or even stand. Finger foods that give a nutritionally adequate diet can be prepared. Foods and drinks can be available any time, day or night.

An additional characteristic of the ideal dementia unit is a practice of discussing terminal care options with the family and, within limits of the law, assisting the family in honoring them. Knowing the family's wishes regarding medical interventions can be a valuable guide. Some states recognize living wills, or a durable power of attorney's right to make decisions for the terminal care of another; others do not. In all cases, families should be intimately involved in these decisions.

Alzheimer's disease is degenerative and eventually terminal. The family should be informed of the natural history of the disease and common decision points in terminal care. A consistent understanding helps staff and family prepare and carry out a plan that is in accord with the resident's values and earlier preferences.

Some families may wish a brain autopsy. Staff assistance in arranging one in advance can help the families prepare for the end. An autopsy offers a definitive diagnosis and may provide satisfaction for a family looking for a meaningful way to contribute to research. Autopsies should be arranged in advance with a research center and locally with a pathologist for removal of the brain. Helping the family work through the details is a joint responsibility between the facility staff and the research center.

Key Outcomes

Numerous positive outcomes are reported from therapeutic programs of caring (see table 1.2). Key outcomes should be measurable and should relate to the characteristics stated above.

On our ideal unit, each resident functions at his or her optimal level. Physical health, weight, and muscle tone are optimally maintained. The quality of social interaction is improved and maintained for a longer period of time into the disease. Family visits are enhanced and fear and grief reduced, through involvement in care planning and implementation. When the time comes, terminal care is appropriate and in accordance with previously discussed plans.

COMMUNICATION AND SUPPORT

Effective communication and mutual support among all persons involved in dementia care are major factors in success. There is almost constant need and opportunity for communication, verbal and nonverbal, and it occurs on many levels.

Staff and Resident

Communication with residents should convey respect, warmth, and acceptance by the staff. These are conveyed by active listening, spoken words, eye contact, facial expressions, touch, and tone of voice.

The staff are taught effective techniques for communication with residents who have impaired language and understanding. For example, instructions are broken down into steps and given one at a time. "Put on your shirt and button it," is a complex procedure for many persons with dementia, unless it is broken into steps that allow sufficient time to complete each one. Even facility staff who have more casual contact with residents are taught to break down thoughts carefully. "Good morning, how are you? What are you doing?" is really three thoughts, demanding at least two answers.

The staff learn to interpret the feelings behind the residents' words or behaviors and are trained to deal with emotional abuse from residents (and sometimes families). For example, staff understand that combative behavior is usually a response to a barrier. Being told (loudly), "No, you can't . . . ," brings resistance. Staff are trained to use soft voices, gentle approaches, and distraction.

Creative listening and interpretation, along with warmth, physical contact, and an opportunity for meaningful repetitive motion are all illustrated in the following exchange between a resident, Helen, and a nursing assistant.

> *Helen:* My mother came back back back . . .
> *N.A.:* Tell me about your mother . . .
> *Helen:* Go to back, go to back, back . . .
> *N.A.:* Did your mother rub your back, like this? (Slowly and gently she rubs Helen's back.)
> *Helen:* (Responds nonverbally by rounding her shoulders, smiling and relaxing. Suddenly, she speaks clearly) We take turns.
> *N.A.:* Oh, would you like to rub my back now?
> *Helen:* (Uses both hands and with a circular motion rubs the nursing assistant's back for several minutes, then gives her a pat.) Go play now!

Staff and Family

The major responsibility for compassionate understanding leading to effective communication lies with the staff, but families can also be gently taught to approach staff with questions and suggestions that bring out cooperation rather than defensiveness. By modeling and by conversation, families are taught better communication skills with their resident family member.

Families may respond angrily or critically out of guilt, grief, or other emotion. Compassion and sensitivity to families' real needs are skills the staff can develop. Families often seek information. Nursing assistants mut be kept informed (e.g., of a resident's medical condition) so that they can give families accurate information. Sharing positive anecdotes about the resident also pleases and encourages families. Staff receptiveness to suggestions from family members also helps them feel an integral part of the team.

Involving families in support groups or arranging for peer support (i.e., facilitating communication between another family member and one who has been through the adjustment period) is another way to extend the process of caring.

Staff and Staff

In addition to the formal system of communication among staff members (care conferences, etc.), the climate for dementia care should encourage informal communication and support. If tensions arise, they must be dealt with quickly, and outside the unit. Residents tend to be sensitive to negative feelings among staff.

In a very small, segregated unit, where there may be one staff person much of the time, the supervisor must ensure that the person does not feel isolated. In a large unit, staff persons must be especially careful to focus on the residents.

Staff and Community

A program of public relations helps the community to understand and be supportive of a dementia program, and to see it as a resource. Such a program might include sponsoring educational meetings open to the public, press releases that report on activities within the unit, a speaker's bureau to address service organizations and other community groups, appearances on talk shows, and donating books on dementia to the local library. Any special media coverage must be closely monitored to protect the privacy and the dignity of residents and their families.

Communication that informs the medical community cannot be neglected. Physicians and home health nurses are often a resident's link to needed services. Sometimes creative methods must be employed to reach these professionals.

Key Outcomes

The positive outcomes of good communication extend to all aspects of nursing home life. This is particularly true in dementia units, where coordination and consistency play key roles in the well-being of residents and their families. Some of the outcomes listed below are also dependent on good training, but it is ongoing communication that allows what was learned in training to be operative.

In our ideal unit, residents are more calm and cooperative, and they respond to these same qualities in staff. Staff and families share reliable information about the resident, and are thus able to meet the resident's needs better. Family visits are enhanced, and families cope better through involvement in care planning and in support groups. Staff are more supportive of each other; turf issues are minimized; and consensus in care planning leads to consistency of approaches. Staff and volunteer recruitment is successful.

Externally, the nursing home and its special dementia programs are viewed in a positive light. The public regards the dementia unit as a resource, and referrals are frequent. As a result, the media use the organization as a source of reliable information about issues relating to dementia.

RESEARCH

The exchange of research findings and clinical experience between the academic community and the providers of care results in continually better guidelines for quality of the dementia residents' life. Applied research is a prerequisite for an enlightened therapeutic approach that minimizes the distress of dementia sufferers and their families.

An organization interested in the highest quality of service affiliates itself, within the limits of its resources, with researchers and associations that advocate or seek answers to the biomedical and psychosocial aspects of dementia care and treatment.

Staff and families generally respond positively to affiliations with credible research institutions. The staff are stimulated by new ideas and become more aware of their efforts. Families and residents have better access to a range of assessment and treatment services.

Involvement in research not only allows the organization, the staff, and families to make a contribution to knowledge; it also brings comfort and hope in the process. As families understand the importance of continued research, they may find altruistic outlets to help work through their grief and loss.

Conclusion

This chapter has presented a philosophy of specialized dementia care based on the concept of a high quality of life and the principles underlying that concept. The application of the principles to special dementia units and programs led to a discussion of practical approaches to the physical environment, selection and training of staff, therapeutic programming, and the important roles of multilevel communication, innovation, and research.

These principles are not ideals. They are derived from experience in the context of developing special dementia programs. We believe these are practical and effective ways to provide quality of life for persons with dementia and for their families. Experience teaches us that the principles may change with new knowledge and understanding.

It is imperative that providers of specialized dementia care consider its impact on the quality of life for the residents. While the progression of the disease cannot be halted, a number of interventions have been found to enhance lives and help ease the emotional burden faced by dementia residents and their families. Perhaps it is this enhancement of human contact, dignity, and comfort that is the greatest benefit of specialized care. We must strive to achieve this for all our demented residents.

Recommended Reading

Berwick, D. 1989. Continuous improvement as an ideal in health care. *New England Journal of Medicine* 320: 53–56.
Belvins, E., Darnell, L., and Bonebrake, C. 1987. *The Nursing Home and You: Part-*

ners in Caring for a Relative with Alzheimer's Disease. Washington, D.C.: American Association of Homes for the Aging.

Freeman, I. 1989. Assuring quality of care in nursing homes: The consumer's role. *Geriatrics* 13: 31–33.

Gwyther, L. P. 1985. *Care of Alzheimer's Patients: A Manual for Nursing Home Staff.* Chicago: Alzheimer's Association.

———— 1988. Nursing home care issues. In M. Aronson (ed.), *Understanding Alzheimer's Disease.* New York: Scribner's.

———— 1989. Selecting a nursing home: Some basic principles help. *Center Reports on Advances in Research* 12: 1–9.

———— 1986. Treating behavior as a symptom of illness. *Provider,* 12(5): 18–21.

Hansen, S. S., Patterson, M. A., and Wilson, R. W. 1988. Family involvement on a dementia unit: The resident enrichment and activity program. *Gerontologist* 28: 508–10.

Kane, R. A. 1989. Toward competent, caring paid caregivers. *Gerontologist* 29: 291–92.

Lemke, S., and Moos, R. 1986. Quality of residential settings for elderly adults. *Journal of Gerontology* 41: 268–76.

Lusky, R. A. 1988. *Research and Education in Alzheimer's Disease and Related Disorders.* Hartford, Conn.: Travelers Center on Aging.

Mace, N. 1987. Programs and services which specialize in the care of persons with dementing illnesses: Issues and options. *American Journal of Alzheimer's Care and Research* 1: 10–17.

———— 1987. Programs and services that specialize in the care of persons with dementia. In *Losing a Million Minds: Confronting the Tragedy of Alzheimer's Disease and Other Dementias.* Washington, D.C.: Congressional Office of Technology Assessment.

Mace, N. L., and Gwyther, L. P. 1989. *Selecting a Nursing Home with a Dedicated Dementia Care Unit.* Chicago: Alzheimer's Association.

McGrowder-Lin, R., and Bhatt, A. 1988. A wanderer's lounge program for nursing home residents with Alzheimer's disease. *Gerontologist* 28: 607–9.

Maslow, K. 1989. *Research Questions for Specialized Nursing Home Care for Persons with Dementia.* Washington, D.C.: Congressional Office of Technology Assessment.

Moss, M. S., and Pfhol, D. C. 1988. New friendships: Staff as visitors of nursing home residents. *Gerontologist* 28: 263–65.

National Citizens Coalition for Nursing Home Reform. 1989. Members urge Pepper Commission to consider current impediments to quality when proposing new programs. *Newsletter* 4: 9–11.

Poer, C. M. 1987. Working with families of residents who have Alzheimer's disease. *Innovations in Long-Term Care* 3: 1–11.

Robinson, A., Spencer, B., and White, L. A. 1988. *Understanding Difficult Behaviors.* Lansing, Mich.: Department of Mental Health.

Shaughnessy, P. W. 1989. Quality of nursing home care. *Generations* 13: 17–20.

Sheridan, C. 1987. *Failure-free activities for the Alzheimer's Patient.* Oakland, Calif.: Cottage Press.

Spalding, J., and Frank, B. W. 1985. Quality care from the resident's point of view. *American Health Care Journal* 11: 3–8.

Tanner, F., Growdon, J. H., and Conner, L. R. (eds.). 1990. *Blueprint for a Specialized Alzheimer's Disease Nursing Home.* Conference proceedings. Boston: Alzheimer's Disease Research Center.

U.S. Congress, Office of Technology Assessment. 1990. Confused Minds, Burdened Families: Finding Help for People with Alzheimer's and Other Dementias. Washington, D.C.: U.S. Government Printing Office.

Wiener, A. S. 1987. A nationwide survey of special units. In Kalicki, A. C. (ed.), *Confronting Alzheimer's Disease.* Owings Mills, Md.: American Association of Homes for the Aging.

2

Care on Dementia Units
in Five States

LAURA J. MATHEW AND PHILIP D. SLOANE

In this chapter, we summarize findings about the process and outcomes of care to cognitively impaired residents of 31 dementia units and 32 comparison units in five states. (Study methods are discussed in the introduction and Appendix.) When appropriate, we present the results of statistical testing. Objective data are supplemented with subjective impressions.

The Physical Appearance of the Residents

Families and visitors entering a nursing home often infer the quality of care residents receive from their personal appearance. The belief of our society that to look good is to feel good is ingrained in many residents themselves. It is not unusual to see the mood of a resident with physical or mental impairment improve when assistance is given to personal appearance and grooming. Consequently, nursing home staff reported that they were often reminded of the importance of providing the best care possible in terms of resident appearance.

Yet grooming can prove difficult in the care of demented persons. Their altered perceptions may cause behavioral outbursts when personal care is given. The nursing staff of dementia units, like others who care for this population, told us they faced this problem on a regular basis. Our study sought to measure their success rate by systematically observing resident grooming in the two settings.

As each resident was observed, we made a judgment about his or her grooming. Three attributes were considered: whether the resident's hair was combed and neat, whether the resident was clean (in terms of remains of food or bodily excretions being present), and whether the resident was dressed neatly and appropriately. We defined neatness of attire not in terms of expensive or fashionable clothing, but in terms of clothing that was not unduly wrinkled or in bad repair. Most forms of clothing were considered appropriate as long as they were clean, fit well, provided adequate protection (e.g., footwear with soles for ambulatory residents), and were appropriate for the setting (especially something other than hospital gowns for residents in public areas).

Each of the three categories of grooming (hair, cleanliness, and dress) was rated on a three-point scale. For example, hair could be rated as excellent, fair, or poor. In two states all ratings were done by the principal investigator. In two other states they were done by a co-investigator. Ratings in the fifth state were completed by either the principal investigator or a research assistant. The three project staff members overlapped in four site visits to ensure reliability of the ratings.

In terms of hair, a higher percentage of dementia unit residents were rated excellent. A total of 227 residents, or 74.7 percent of all those observed on dementia units, were in this category. On the comparison units, 56.1 percent of all the residents observed were rated excellent. Table 2.1 displays this finding. The differences were significant (chi-square with 2 degrees of freedom = 23.6, $p < .01$).

Similar results were obtained in terms of dress and cleanliness. A total of 237, or 78.2 percent, dementia unit residents observed were rated excellent for dress. This is contrasted to 187 (60.1 percent) comparison unit residents. The differences were significant (chi-square with 2 degrees of freedom = 24.8, $p < .05$). In terms of cleanliness, 268 (88.4 percent) dementia unit residents observed were rated excellent, and 233 (74.4 percent) of comparison unit residents observed were in this category. Again, the differences were significant (chi-square with 2 degrees of freedom = 20.1, $p < .05$). We conclude that although caring only for cognitively impaired residents, the dementia units provided care that was notably better as judged from resident appearance.

TABLE 2.1   Rating of Personal Care Given to Residents

Area Observed	Dementia Unit Residents (N = 304)	Comparison Unit Residents (N = 314)	p
Hair care			
Good	74.7%	56.1%	<.01
Fair	22.0	38.5	
Poor	3.3	5.4	
Neatness of clothing			
Good	78.2	60.1	<.01
Fair	19.8	33.8	
Poor	2.0	6.1	
Overall cleanliness			
Good	88.5	74.4	<.01
Fair	11.2	24.3	
Poor	0.3	1.3	

Prevalence of Broken Skin

As in many health care settings, the occurrence of decubitus and other broken skin are problematic for nursing homes. The nursing staff make continuing efforts to address this issue, most of them preventive. Turning or ambulating residents with limitations in movement are common practices. In the best of circumstances, these practices may not always succeed either because of lapses in caregiving or because of resident factors such as severe illness or resistance to caregivers.

We attempted to measure the success of preventing broken skin by obtaining data on the number of residents being treated for decubitus. Specifically, we documented the number of residents with stage 2 to stage 4 pressure sores or open skin tears. Our source of data was the charge nurse for the units we visited. When questions arose regarding severity of the decubitus, records on decubitus care were consulted.

We found that 37 residents on dementia units were being treated for stage 2 to stage 4 decubitus or other broken skin areas. Since the dementia units housed 965 residents, these 37 residents represented 3.8 percent of all dementia unit residents. Likewise, we noted 115 (of a total of 1,883) comparison unit residents being treated for stage 2 to stage 4 pressure sores or other broken skin areas. They represented 6.1 percent of all residents on the comparison units. This difference was statistically significant (chi-square with 1 degree of freedom = 6.53, $p < .05$). These results are displayed in table 2.2. Since the dementia residents on the com-

TABLE 2.2   Residents Treated for Pressure Sores (%)

	Dementia Unit Residents ($N = 965$)	Comparison Unit Residents ($N = 1883$)
Residents without skin breakdown	96.2	93.9
Residents under treatment	3.8	6.1

Note: $p < .05$.

parison units were more physically impaired than those on the dementia units (see introduction and chapter 4), we cannot infer whether the lower decubitus rate in dementia units is due to resident factors or to care practices.

Weight Loss Among Residents

Providing adequate nutrition to victims of dementia can be problematic. The cognitively impaired resident may have difficulty recognizing and communicating a sense of hunger (Mace and Rabins 1981). Furthermore, the disease process itself may result in a loss of weight and muscle mass, even when adequate amounts of food are taken. Awareness of the importance of nutrition for demented residents is essential.

During the review of medical records, we documented the current weights of residents in our sample. In addition, we noted the weight of each resident three months before our visit. We were able to obtain this data on a total of 537 residents; the other residents' medical records did not have complete information on weight. In addition, some residents had been in the units for less than three months, and prior weights were unobtainable.

Our data are grouped by gender and setting (dementia unit or comparison unit). In table 2.3, residents are divided into four categories based on their weight three months before our site visit. These categories were estimates we arrived at by consensus. A limitation of the study is that the data categories do not consider ideal body weight for the residents. The heights and body frames of the residents were not recorded. Thus, we were unable to place residents in a precise category based on their ideal body weight. As a result, too many residents were probably placed in the "adequate" or "questionable" categories.

Nonetheless, our data delineate the number of female and male demented residents who were losing weight in both settings. Few differences were apparent. Taking both the inadequate and questionable categories into consideration, 54 female residents lost weight in the com-

TABLE 2.3 Weight Change Patterns during the Three Months
before the Site Visit

Initial Weight Status	Dementia Units			Comparison Units		
	Gained Weight	Remained Stable	Lost Weight	Gained Weight	Remained Stable	Lost Weight
Women						
Inadequate (≤90 lb.)	18	5	8	2	7	4
Questionable (91–130 lb.)	42	37	60	38	36	50
Adequate (131–160 lb.)	12	14	20	22	11	19
Overweight (>160 lb.)	7	1	6	1	2	5
Men						
Inadequate (≤110 lb.)	0	3	0	1	1	1
Questionable (111–150 lb.)	7	3	11	12	8	15
Adequate (151–184 lb.)	4	2	13	6	3	12
Overweight (>184 lb.)	2	2	2	0	0	2

Note: The table shows numbers of study subjects.

parison units, compared with 68 residents in the dementia units. A total of 16 male residents in these two categories lost weight in the comparison unit, as opposed to 11 male residents from the dementia units. Neither of these differences was statistically significant.

We conclude that there were few differences in weight loss for the residents overall. Reasons for this could include a lack of sensitivity in our instrumentation, since most nursing home records do not provide enough information to estimate ideal body weight. There is also a probability that the similarity in weight loss for both settings was related in the fact that all residents in our sample were demented. The type of care provided may not have affected the ability to improve nutrition, although this theory is difficult to test within the limitations of this project.

Planned Activities Offered in Each Setting

The need to involve demented residents in therapeutic activity has been well documented (Burnside 1984, Coons and Weaverdyck 1986,

McArthur 1988). Such activity is varied and includes time spent with someone on a one-to-one basis, as well as time spent in small groups. Programs offered by nursing homes assist residents by improving physical and mental skills and may include activities such as exercise or reminiscence therapy. Individualized programs include sessions on personal grooming or attempts at obtaining better bowel and bladder control.

Our questionnaires completed by administrative staff of the units we visited included a checklist of different services known to be offered in long-term care settings. We asked the staff completing the questionnaire to indicate which services were currently being provided for the residents of their units. Table 2.4 lists these services by type of setting. For each service category, units could respond that the service was not available, available but had to be chosen for a particular resident, or provided to all residents.

Almost no differences were seen between the dementia units and the comparison units in terms of services offered. Of all the services, only mental status testing showed a statistically significant difference. Dementia units were more likely to offer this to all residents (chi-square with 2 degrees of freedom = 14.19, $p < .01$). Dementia units showed a trend to provide more services to families of demented residents, but the difference was not statistically significant (chi-square with 2 degrees of freedom = 4.98, $p = .08$). All other responses were similar for the two types of setting.

We conclude that the range of services reported to be available to demented residents of nursing homes does not differ between dementia units and comparison units. Reasons for this may include the following: (1) Our sample of dementia units may represent facilities that do not emphasize the importance of activity for their residents. (2) While the need for activity programming has been well documented, it has not been fully researched. Thus, there may still be some reluctance to begin a service without prior knowledge about its potential. (3) Our dementia units were on the average less than five years old. This early stage may mean that a fully developed therapeutic milieu is yet to evolve among all dementia units. That is, while some policies and procedures, such as the use of restraints, may be well defined, the practice of providing activities may not be universally observed. (4) We asked only about service availability. We did not gather information on the quality or intensity of services provided. Thus, our questionnaire may not have been sensitive to the way services are offered.

Other types of activities that were not on our checklist were offered. These were recorded through our subjective notes. They include the following special activities offered on some dementia units: music activities, such as sing-alongs or a rhythm band; eating activities, such as ice

TABLE 2.4   Availability of Various Services

Service	No.	(%) of Dementia Units	No.	(%) of Comparison Units
Individual care plan				
Not available	0	(0)	0	(0)
Available	1	(3.3)	1	(3.1)
All residents receive	29	(96.7)	31	(96.9)
Mental status testing				
Not available	4	(13.3)	16	(51.6)*
Available	7	(23.3)	9	(29.0)
All residents receive	19	(63.3)	6	(19.4)
Functional assessment				
Not available	1	(3.3)	3	(9.7)
Available	5	(16.7)	8	(25.8)
All residents receive	24	(80.0)	20	(64.5)
Physical therapy				
Not available	1	(3.3)	0	(0)
Available	25	(83.3)	28	(87.5)
All residents receive	4	(13.3)	4	(12.5)
Occupational therapy				
Not available	2	(6.9)	3	(9.4)
Available	23	(79.3)	25	(78.1)
All residents receive	4	(13.8)	4	(12.5)
Reality orientation				
Not available	0	(0)	1	(3.2)
Available	9	(32.1)	18	(58.1)
All residents receive	19	(67.9)	12	(38.7)
Activities program				
Not available	0	(0)	0	(0)
Available	3	(10.0)	3	(9.4)
All residents receive	27	(90.0)	29	(90.6)
Individual bladder training				
Not available	0	(0)	2	(6.3)
Available	18	(64.3)	25	(78.1)
All residents receive	10	(35.7)	5	(15.6)
Programs for families				
Not available	6	(20.0)	13	(44.8)
Available	13	(43.3)	11	(37.9)
All residents receive	11	(36.7)	5	(17.2)
Individual mobility program				
Not available	3	(10.7)	2	(6.7)
Available	18	(64.3)	18	(60.0)
All residents receive	7	(25.0)	10	(33.3)

(*continued*)

TABLE 2.4   (*Continued*)

Service	No.	(%) of Dementia Units	No.	(%) of Comparison Units
Assistance in self-care				
Not available	0	(0)	4	(12.9)*
Available	9	(30.0)	19	(61.3)
All residents receive	21	(70.0)	8	(25.8)
Reminiscence group				
Not available	3	(10.0)	4	(13.3)**
Available	10	(33.3)	20	(66.7)
All residents receive	17	(56.7)	6	(20.0)
Reading group				
Not available	2	(7.4)	2	(6.7)
Available	15	(55.6)	23	(76.7)
All residents receive	10	(37.0)	5	(16.7)

Note: For some services the numbers do not add up to 62 because information is missing.
*Indicates significance of a chi-square statistic at .01.
**Indicates significance at .05.

cream socials; dance therapy; humorous movies; riding excursions in a bus or van; folding laundry; beauty shop; pet therapy; bowling with plastic balls and pins; group exercises using a large parachute; baking; woodcraft; gardening; religious services; and cocktail parties.

Dementia unit staff often agreed that television hindered most types of interaction; only nondemented residents are actually able to enjoy most television programs. In addition, staff often commented on the need to individualize the activities for residents according to their needs and said that even the hard-to-reach resident was able to benefit from activities if enough creativity and thought went into planning. Last, staff commented on the need for joint planning among all disciplines working with the resident; this seemed to work best through the use of multi-disciplinary rounds.

Location and Interaction among Residents and Staff

Dementia units, like many therapeutic settings, are designed to promote interaction among the residents. Staff members often attempt to maintain or improve verbal or nonverbal communication skills. Staff also attempt to keep the residents out of their rooms during much of the day, to encourage interaction and sensory stimulation, and to prevent too much daytime sleeping (and the nighttime wakefulness that often results). Because of the emphasis on engaging residents in meaningful dialogue and activity, we tried to identify and describe the effectiveness of this process. This was made possible through our observations of the residents, which documented their location and levels of interaction during two types of daytime observations.

We defined location in terms of being either in a public area (i.e., a day room, hallway, dining room) or a private area (i.e., the resident's own room or bathroom). We defined interaction as some type of active involvement with others. To be actively involved, the resident had to show some signs of participating in a group activity, being physically assisted by a staff member or other person, or speaking or interacting in some fashion with another person. Specifically, for residents in public areas, six conditions were possible. Residents could either be sitting and not participating, sitting and passively participating, sitting and actively participating, standing or walking alone, standing or walking with others, or in an "other" category. For residents in their own rooms, nine conditions were possible. Residents could be in bed alone, in bed with staff attending, in bed interacting with a roommate or visitors, out of bed alone or not interacting, out of bed with staff attending, out of bed interacting with a roommate or visitors, in the bathroom alone, in the bathroom assisted, or in an "other" category.

In addition to 10 residents chosen at random, we also gathered observational data on the unit as a whole. In this manner, we were able to describe the location of all residents and staff, their activity level, the number of residents and staff actually interacting, and other aspects of the environment.

A possible source of error in this unit observation data is the percentage of the unit census that was actually observed (see table 2.6). During the unit observations, we were not able to count all residents. If residents were in their own rooms behind closed doors, we did not enter their rooms. Other residents of a unit may have been off the unit during our observations. We noted the census of every unit we visited and the total number of residents observed. This allowed us to ascertain the proportion of residents observed. We were able to observe more residents on dementia units than on comparison units.

LOCATION AND INTERACTION LEVELS OF RESIDENTS IN SAMPLE

When we observed our sample of 10 residents chosen at random from each unit, we attempted to be as unobtrusive as possible. We asked for assistance from one staff member, who identified residents for us. The observation times avoided meals and shift changes.

TABLE 2.5   Residents in Public and Private Areas

	In Public Areas	In Private Areas	p
Sample residents			
Dementia unit sample[a] (N = 302)	69.9%	30.1%	<.01
Comparison unit sample[a] (N = 313)	39.0	61.0	
All unit residents			
On dementia units[b] (N = 803)	75.1	24.9	<.01
On comparison units[b] (N = 1428)	40.9	59.1	

[a]The actual sample size was 307 dementia unit residents and 318 comparison unit residents, but it was not possible to observe all of them.
[b]The percentage of the unit census actually observed was 83.2 for the dementia units and 75.8 for the comparison units.

On dementia units, we found that 69.9 percent, or 211 of 302 residents observed, were out of their rooms. This was contrasted to 39 percent, or 122 of all 313 residents observed on the comparison units. Table 2.5 lists these differences in resident location. Dementia unit residents were more likely to be out of their own rooms and in a public area, and the difference was statistically significant (chi-square with 1 degree of freedom = 59.1, $p < .01$).

One finding of interest was in the number of residents found alone and in bed. This single category provided insight into the dissimilarity of the two settings. A total of 93 residents on comparison units, or 29.7 percent of the 302 persons observed in our sample, were in this category. On the dementia units, 42 persons, or 13.9 percent of the 313 persons in our sample, were in bed alone.

When we walked through the units, systematically observing all residents not behind closed doors, we again found differences in the two types of settings. In terms of location of residents on the dementia units, 603 residents (75.1 percent) were found in public areas and 200 residents (24.9 percent) were in their own rooms. On the comparison units, a total of 584 (40.9 percent) residents were found in public areas and 844 (59.1 percent) residents were in their own rooms. The figures for comparison units include nondemented residents, and were remarkably similar to the sample of demented residents. Thus, this method of observation also found a higher proportion of residents out of their rooms on dementia

TABLE 2.6   Involvement of Residents in Interaction

	Involved	Not Involved	p
Dementia unit sample (N = 302)	37.0%	63.0%	< .01
Comparison unit sample (N = 313)	23.0	77.0	
All residents observed on dementia units (N = 803)	31.9	68.1	< .01
All residents observed on comparison units (N = 1428)	19.25	80.75	

units than on the comparison units. Table 2.5 displays the proportions of all residents in public and private areas by type of setting. Again the difference is statistically significant (chi-square with 1 degree of freedom = 241.9, p < .01).

Our observations also found that more dementia unit residents were involved in some type of interaction, either in public areas or in their own rooms. A total of 302 residents on dementia units were observed during our resident sample observations; 37 percent (112 residents) were actively participating in some form of interaction. In contrast, of 313 residents observed on the comparison units, 23 percent (73 residents) were actively participating. Conversely, the number of residents who were found alone or not involved in any form of interaction was higher in the comparison units. A total of 240 residents, or 77 percent of our comparison unit sample, were not interacting. This was compared with 190 residents, or 63 percent, of our dementia unit sample. Table 2.6 displays these differences. The differences were significant (chi-square with 1 degree of freedom = 13.8, p < .01), indicating that more dementia unit residents were involved in some form of interaction than comparison unit residents.

Results were similar when we made our walk-through unit observations (table 2.6). On the dementia units, 31.9 percent of the residents were involved in some interaction, and 68.1 percent were not involved. While 31.9 percent of the entire dementia unit population does not represent a majority, the proportion of dementia unit residents interacting was higher than on the comparison units. About 19.25 percent of the residents on comparison units were involved in some interaction, and 80.75 percent were not involved. The difference was again statistically significant (chi-square with 1 degree of freedom = 44.9, $p < .01$). Thus, as was seen with resident location, a higher proportion of residents interacted on the dementia units than on the comparison units.

Considering that the comparison unit population observed included demented and nondemented residents, and the dementia unit population included only demented residents (whose communication skills are impaired), one would expect the proportion of residents observed in some form of interaction to be higher on the comparison units. That is, the nondemented residents (with more ability to communicate) on the comparison units would increase the likelihood that interaction would occur in these settings. However, this is not what we found. Even with the limitations of caring only for demented residents, the dementia units had a higher proportion of residents involved in some form of interaction.

INTERACTION LEVEL OF UNIT STAFF

To assess the degree of staff involvement in activities that entailed direct contact with residents, we observed staff-resident interactions. A total of 213 staff members were observed during a morning or afternoon walk-through on the 31 dementia units involved in the study. Of these, 41.9 percent were observed in some form of activity that involved direct interaction with the residents. A total of 343 staff members were observed on the 32 comparison units in the study. Of these, 35.6 percent were observed in some form of interaction that involved residents. A higher proportion of staff on the comparison units (64.4 percent versus 57.3 percent on the dementia units) was observed performing duties that did not directly involve residents. Table 2.7 presents the differences in staff involvement by type of setting. Staff involvement in direct contact with residents tended to be higher on the dementia units than on the comparison units, but the differences did not reach a statistically significant level (chi-square with 1 degree of freedom = 2.85, $p < .092$).

In conclusion, we noted significant differences in the two settings in terms of resident location and resident interaction levels. This was true not only for our sample but for all residents we observed. Dementia units had a higher amount of interaction, and residents were more often out of their rooms participating in some event. Staff on the dementia units tended to interact more with the residents, but the difference was not as great as the residents' overall levels of interaction and did not reach statistical significance.

This finding is in contrast to the previous section of this chapter, which reported virtually no differences between the two settings in regard to planned activities. It supports the hypothesis that the list of

TABLE 2.7   Contact of Staff with Residents (%)

	Dementia Unit Staff Observed ($N = 213$)	Comparison Unit Staff Observed ($N = 343$)
In direct contact with residents	42.7	35.6
Not in direct contact with residents	57.3	64.4

Note: $p = .092$.

services does not differ, but actual time spent in direct human contact is greater on the dementia units. Certainly, dementia unit proponents emphasize the importance of contact between residents and staff. This emphasis was visible and clearly noted during some unit observations.

Mobility Status of Residents

The aging process is associated with physiological changes and chronic conditions that can discourage the elderly from some forms of exercise. These factors at times lead to impairment of mobility. The dementias amplify this problem as disease progression tends to produce difficulties in ambulation. Consequently, a basic nursing function is to promote the resident's maximum possible level of physical activity.

Because we believe that good nursing care for the demented person requires consideration of this issue, we studied the mobility status of the residents. Once again the abilities of residents on the dementia units were compared with those of residents on comparison units. For this procedure, we used data on resident mobility as (1) reported by the staff using the Multidimensional Observational Scale for Elderly Subjects (MOSES), and (2) noted during our own observations of residents.

ABILITY TO AMBULATE AS REPORTED BY STAFF

The MOSES instrument was completed for each resident by either a nurse or a nursing assistant who knew the resident's functional status. The MOSES assesses mobility by asking whether the resident: walks without any assistance, moves independently with mechanical assistance, walks with physical assistance of staff, or remains bedfast or chairfast.

By this measure, residents of the dementia units had more ability to ambulate than those receiving traditional care. Table 2.8 lists the percentages in each category for both settings. A total of 60.5 percent of dementia unit residents were able to walk without any assistance, as compared to

TABLE 2.8   Ability of Residents to Ambulate as Reported by Staff Members (%)

	Dementia Unit Residents ($N = 306$)	Comparison Unit Residents ($N = 318$)
Walks without assistance	60.5	19.5
Walks independently with mechanical device	9.8	20.2
Walks with physical assistance	16.0	16.9
Is bedfast or chairfast	13.7	43.4

Note: $p < .01$.

19.5 percent of residents receiving traditional care. A higher percentage (43.4) of residents on comparison units were bedfast or chairfast; dementia units had only 13.7 percent in this category. The differences are statistically significant (chi-square with 3 degrees of freedom = 124.8, $p < .01$), with residents on dementia units described as having more ability to ambulate than those on comparison units.

ABILITY TO AMBULATE AS OBSERVED DURING VISITS

Our observation form listed five options for describing mobility status. Residents could either be ambulating, in bed, in a wheelchair, in a geri-chair, or in some other chair.

Table 2.9 displays the observed mobility status of residents in both settings. Dementia unit residents were more often observed walking and were less likely to be in bed. The differences were statistically significant (chi-square with 4 degrees of freedom = 101.5, $p < .01$).

Further analysis attempted to determine a more accurate number of residents who were actually mobile (besides those we observed walking around) on the units. Because no additional observational information was available, we could not determine the true mobility status of residents in bed, in a wheelchair, or in a geri-chair. However, we surmised that residents in some other chair, such as a recliner or sofa, must have walked (with or without assistance) to that location and thus inferred that they were ambulatory. Therefore we included as "mobile" residents we observed walking around and those sitting in a chair other than a wheelchair or geri-chair. A total of 86 residents (27.4 percent) observed on the comparison units were "mobile." In contrast, 206 (67.8 percent) dementia unit residents were "mobile." These findings were consistent with staff reports from the MOSES, indicating that residents on dementia units were more mobile.

TABLE 2.9   Mobility of Residents during a Single Daytime Observation (%)

	Dementia Unit Residents ($N = 304$)	Comparison Unit Residents ($N = 314$)
Walking	35.2	13.4
In bed	14.5	30.6
In wheelchair	12.8	31.2
In geri-chair	4.9	10.8
In other chair	32.6	14.0

Note: $p < .01$.

PREDICTING MOBILITY STATUS

The results reported above do not control for other factors that can influence mobility, such as the possibility that dementia unit residents were in an earlier stage of disease than comparison unit residents. In an attempt to control for such factors, we next used a multivariate statistical technique, logistic regression. Our outcome variable was the ambulatory status of the residents ("mobile" versus "nonmobile"). That is, we explored the relationship of several factors to the mobility of residents. The exposure variable (which represented the treatment in question) was the type of setting (dementia unit or comparison unit). Nine independent variables (potential confounders) were part of the model. These were all resident characteristics. The variables tested were: diagnoses known to affect mobility (such as arthritis, stroke, hip fracture, and cardiovascular disease), age of the resident, frequency of family visits, length of time since first admission to a nursing home, type of payment, race, sex, behavior problems (based on the MOSES instrument), and number of medications taken.

The final model identified four factors that affect the relationship between type of setting and mobility; the other factors tested were not associated with mobility status. The four confounders were the resident's age, the length of time since the first nursing home admission, the number of medications taken, and the type of payment. Of these, type of setting, resident age, and length of time since first nursing home admission had the strongest associations with mobility status. Controlling for these factors, the odds that the resident's observed status would be ambulatory remained four to five times greater for residents on the dementia units than for residents receiving traditional care (odds ratio [O.R.] = 4.64, 95 percent confidence interval = 3.24, 6.65).

Based on these analyses, we conclude that residents on dementia units are more mobile than residents on comparison units. Even when resident characteristics such as age, stage of illness (estimated using length of stay in a nursing home), or affliction with diseases known to affect mobility are considered, residence on a dementia unit is associated with a higher chance of being mobile. The reasons for this association cannot be determined form our data. Two alternative explanations are possible. Either other factors (such as mobility status on admission, or dementia unit discharge policies) caused these differences and were not adequately controlled for, or dementia units are preventing immobility (for example, by restraining less and encouraging activity).

Use of Medications

Nursing home residents often receive numerous daily medications. Studies have shown that nursing home residents can be subject to over-prescribing by physicians and to clinical misuse by nurses who too frequently turn to medications as a response to symptoms (LeSage 1982). Our study sought to describe and compare the use of routinely administered medications by residents in dementia and comparison units.

Information collected on site visits included a complete list of medications currently administered on a routine basis, including vitamins, laxatives, and topical medications. Dosages were not recorded except for psychotropic medications, for which the total daily dose was recorded. PRN drugs were not included because such drugs comprise only a small proportion of total drugs used.

TOTAL NUMBER OF MEDICATIONS

The total number of regularly prescribed medications received by the dementia unit residents ranged from 0 to 14, with a mean of 3.30. For residents on comparison units, the range was 0 to 12, with a mean of 4.16. The difference in the means is statistically significant ($t = 4.61$, $p < .01$).

The percentages of residents receiving specific numbers of total medications are plotted on figure 2.1. More dementia unit residents are found in categories receiving fewer total medications. Percentages of comparison unit residents are higher in categories corresponding to greater numbers of medications. Thus comparison unit residents, or those receiving traditional care, seem to receive significantly more total medications than the residents on dementia units.

MAJOR MEDICATION USE

We then excluded "minor" medications—those unlikely to cause serious adverse affects. These minor medications included vitamins, lax-

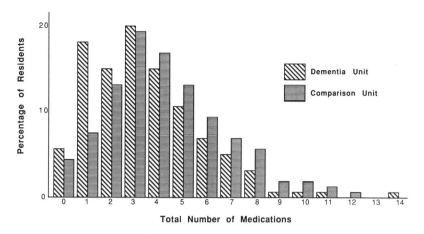

FIGURE 2.1   Percentage of residents in each setting and total number of medications being administered.

atives, and topicals. What remained we called major medications. The range of these major medications for dementia unit residents was 0 to 8, with a mean of 2.32. For residents on the comparison units, the range was 0 to 9, with a mean of 2.81. The difference in the means was again statistically significant ($t = 3.25$, $p < .01$). Thus, even when the influence of minor drugs such as vitamins and laxatives is deleted, residents on the comparison units still received more medications than their counterparts on the dementia units.

PRESCRIBING PATTERNS OF INDIVIDUAL UNITS

We next explored the prescribing patterns for individual dementia and comparison units. In this analysis, the mean numbers of medications received by subjects in each of the 63 units were studied. We looked for differences in prescribing patterns by state, by ownership status (for profit and nonprofit), and by level of care. Two facilities (one comparison unit in Texas and one comparison unit in North Carolina) were outliers in terms of overall prescribing. These two facilities tended to medicate residents much more than others. Overall, however, no statistically significant effect of state, ownership, or level of care was found. Thus, the differences we observed between dementia and comparison units appear to represent a general trend rather than increased prescribing in a few comparison units.

THE EFFECT OF RESIDENT AGE ON DRUG USE

We next sought to determine if the differences we observed in prescribing rates were due to differences in the characteristics of residents in the two settings. The first characteristic we explored was resident age. The mean numbers of major medications given in each of the 31 dementia units and the 32 comparison units were plotted against 10 age groups. The age groups consisted of equally spaced five-year intervals beginning at 51 years of age and ending at 100 years. There was no statistically significant linear association between age and the number of major medications taken. However, there was a statistically significant pattern for the age group from 75 to 85 years to receive more major medications than either the youngest age group (less than 75 years old) or the oldest (over 85). This pattern was present in both dementia and comparison units, however; so age did not appear to contribute to the differences observed between the two settings.

CATEGORIES OF MEDICATIONS

Next, we studied patterns of prescribing by type of medication. Twelve categories of drugs were used: topical medications, ophthalmological ointments and drops, vitamins and supplements, potassium, laxatives and stool softeners, analgesics, major tranquilizers, minor tranquilizers and hypnotics, antidepressants, combination tranquilizer-antidepressant drugs, cardiovascular or vasodilating drugs, and an "other" category. The "other" category included a wide variety of medications, such as those given for Parkinson's disease or cancer. Hypnotics were administered infrequently; for this reason they were grouped in the related category of minor tranquilizers. Figure 2.2 shows the percentage of residents in each setting taking specific categories of medications. We found statistically significant differences in only four categories of drugs: cardiovascular or vasodilating drugs, vitamins, laxatives, and potassium. Residents on comparison units received each of these types of mediations more often than residents on dementia units. Differences in the prescribing patterns for the other eight categories of medications were not statistically significant.

PSYCHOTROPIC MEDICATIONS

Because reduction in psychotropic medications is a goal of many dementia units (Weiner 1987), we examined in detail the use of these drugs. In our combined sample, the 10 most widely prescribed drugs in descending order of use were: haloperidol (Haldol), thioridazine (Mellaril), diphenhydramine (Benadryl), amitriptyline (Elavil), alprazolam (Xanax), chlorpromazine (Thorazine), lorazepam (Ativan), temaze-

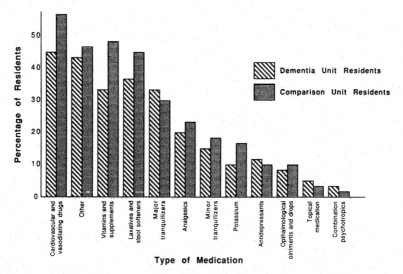

FIGURE 2.2 Percentage of residents in each setting taking each category of medication.

TABLE 2.10 Use of Psychotropic Medications (%)

	Dementia Unit Residents ($N = 307$)	Comparison Unit Residents ($N = 318$)
Haloperidol (Haldol)	17.3	14.5
Thioridazine (Mellaril)	12.1	12.0
Diphenhydramine (Benadryl)	2.9	4.4
Amitriptyline (Elavil)	2.9	1.9
Alprazolam (Xanax)	2.3	3.1
Chlorpromazine (Thorazine)	2.0	1.6
Lorazepam (Ativan)	1.6	2.8
Tamazepam (Restoril)	1.3	1.9
Triazolam* (Halcion)	0.7	3.1
Doxepin* (Sinequan)	0.3	4.1

*Statistically significant differences ($p < .05$).

pam (Restoril), triazolam (Halcion), and doxepin (Sinequan). Other major and minor tranquilizers, antidepressants, and hypnotics were occasionally found in the records, but each was administered to fewer than 10 residents.

Table 2.10 lists the 10 most frequently prescribed psychotropic medications and the percentage of residents in each type of setting taking them. Although a higher percentage of dementia unit residents took haloperidol, amitriptyline, and chlorpromazine by comparison with residents receiving traditional care, the difference was not statistically significant. Only in the case of doxepin and triazolam were statistically significant differences found; residents on comparison units received a higher amount of these drugs. Because of the small number of residents involved and the large number of significance tests performed, however, we doubt that these differences represent a clinically meaningful finding.

When all psychotropic medications were grouped together, no statistically significant difference was noted between dementia and comparison units. Fifty percent of all dementia unit residents received no psychotropics, compared to 52 percent of residents on comparison units (chi-square with 1 degree of freedom = 0.26, $p < .61$).

DAILY DOSAGES OF HALOPERIDOL AND THIORIDAZINE

Having demonstrated no difference in overall prescribing, we next sought to determine if the dosages used by dementia units were lower. In this analysis, we examined the average daily dose of haloperidol (Haldol) and thioridazine (Mellaril). These were the two most commonly used psychotropic agents, and we had enough subjects on these drugs to make meaningful comparisons.

Fifty-two residents on dementia units took haloperidol. The total daily dose ranged from 0.5 mg to 21 mg; the mean daily dose was 2.28 mg. Forty-five residents on comparison units were taking haloperidol. The total daily dose here ranged from 0.5 mg to 35 mg; the mean daily dose for these residents was 2.80 mg. When the means in total daily dosage were tested, the difference was not statistically significant ($t = -0.58$, $p = .57$).

Similar results were found in the use of thioridazine. Thirty-seven residents on dementia units received this drug. The total daily dose ranged from 10 mg to 300 mg, and the mean total daily dose was 57.7 mg. The comparison units had 38 residents who took this drug; total daily dose ranged from 10 mg to 300 mg, and the mean total daily dose was 64.6 mg. Once again, when the means were compared, there was no statistically significant difference ($t = -0.46$, $p = .64$).

In summary, there does not seem to be a difference in the prescribing patterns for haloperidol and thioridazine between the two settings. Both dementia and comparison units administer these drugs and use them similarly.

PREDICTORS OF MULTIPLE MEDICATION USE

As noted above, our initial comparisons showed that dementia unit residents received fewer medications than comparison unit residents. Without further analysis, however, we would not know if this finding represented differences in care between the two settings or was the result of other factors. For example, comparison unit residents might receive more medications because they have more illnesses requiring mediations.

To address this problem, we attempted to control for resident and facility differences that might contribute to the medication-prescribing differences we observed between dementia units and comparison units. This analysis used logistic regression, a statistical technique that allows for simultaneous control of multiple variables.

The outcome variable was the number of major medications administered to the residents. As explained before, this involved omitting minor medications such as vitamins. Specifically, the outcome of interest in this procedure was whether a resident was taking three or more, as opposed to two or fewer, major medications. The exposure variable (which represented the treatment in question) was the type of setting. This could either be a dementia unit or a comparison unit.

Ten independent variables (or potential confounders) were studied. The variables tested were: the number of diagnoses likely to require medication (such as diabetes, hypertension, cardiac disease, glaucoma, and arthritis), the age of the resident, the frequency of family visits, the length of time since first admission to a nursing home, the type of payment, race, sex, behavior problems (based on the MOSES instrument), activities of daily living (ADL) impairment score, and the state. An interaction term involving the type of setting and the state was also included, so that we could explore differences among the units in the five different states.

Four variables were found to be independent predictors of major medication use. These were the number of serious diseases generally requiring medication, the type of setting (dementia unit or comparison unit), the age of the resident, and the state. Of these four, the most highly significant factor is the number of serious diseases; type of setting is the second most important.

The odds of taking more than two major medications is roughly one and one-half times greater for residents in the comparison units than those in the dementia units (O.R. = 1.648, 95 percent confidence interval:

1.135, 2.391). Adjusting for the facility characteristic of state and the resident characteristics of age, race, sex, length of time since first admission to a nursing home, number of diseases likely to result in medications, behavior problems, ADL score, frequency of family visits, and type of payment did not have an appreciable effect on the magnitude of this association.

We conclude that residents on the comparison units were administered a greater number of medications overall. This was the case even when we controlled for other factors that might explain higher medication rates in comparison units. Thus, the traditional nursing home setting may involve policies or procedures that result in a higher tendency to medicate dementia residents. In contrast, dementia units use fewer medications.

Use of Restraints

As we began planning the project, experts in the field often told us that a dementia unit symbolized freedom from physical and chemical restraints. Because of the many practical and ethical problems associated with restraining the elderly, this benefit alone seemed to justify the establishment of a unit. Thus we sought to measure the practice of restraining and to study its effect.

USE OF PHYSICAL RESTRAINTS AS REPORTED BY STAFF

The MOSES instrument included an item asking whether the resident was physically restrained during the previous week. Staff completing this item had four possible responses: not at all, seldom, at times, or often. Definitions of these terms are provided on the MOSES so that responses are consistent. For example, "seldom" is defined as "on one to three days (during the past week) for only short periods of time," and often is defined as "on more than three days (during the past week) for most of the day."

Table 2.11 compares the results for the two sets of residents. Dementia unit residents exceed the comparison unit residents in the "not at all" category; 55.4 percent of dementia unit residents and 27.4 percent of comparison unit residents were in this category. The comparison unit residents exceed the dementia unit residents in the "often" category. The differences were statistically significant (chi-square with 3 degrees of freedom = 70.91, $p < .01$).

TABLE 2.11   Use of Physical Restraints as Reported by Staff Members (%)

	Dementia Unit Residents (N = 305)	Comparison Unit Residents (N = 318)
Not at all	55.4	27.4
Seldom	8.2	5.3
At times	9.5	7.5
Often	26.9	59.8

Note: $p < .01$.

USE OF PHYSICAL RESTRAINT ON RESIDENTS OUT OF BED: SITE VISIT OBSERVATIONS

As we visited each unit, we briefly observed all study subjects during an unannounced walk-through. At that time, we noted whether the resident was up walking, in bed, in a wheelchair, in a geri-chair, or in some other chair. We also documented whether or not the resident was physically tied down (e.g., with wrist restraints, posey belts, or a sheet tied behind a chair).

For analysis purposes, we defined physical restraints as present if a person was tied to a chair or was sitting in a geri-chair. The geri-chair has a large table in front of the seated person. This table forms a type of restraint because it can only be removed by a person other than the one seated in the chair. It is nearly impossible for residents in geri-chairs to move elsewhere on their own volition. Consequently, all residents found in geri-chairs were included among those who were restrained. We did not include in this analysis any people who were in bed when observed because (1) we were ambivalent about whether bed rails constitute a restraint, and (2) we were primarily interested in restraint use when individuals were out of bed.

Table 2.12 displays our findings. A total of 70.1 percent of residents on dementia units were not restrained during our observations, and 15.5 percent were restrained. This gave us a grand total of 260 residents (85.6 percent of the sample) on dementia units to include for the analysis. A total of 33.5 percent of the residents of comparison units were not restrained, and 36.1 percent were restrained. Comparison unit residents thus totaled 219 (69.9 percent of the sample) for this analysis. The differences were significant (chi-square with 5 degrees of freedom = 87.0, $p <$ .01); the comparison units physically restrained residents more often.

Our observations of the residents were brief and were made only

TABLE 2.12   Physical Restraint Status during a Single Daytime Observation (%)

Status	Dementia Unit Residents (N = 304)	Comparison Unit Residents (N = 314)
In bed	14.5	30.6
Out of bed		
Restrained		
Tied to a chair	10.5	25.2
In geri-chair		
Tied	2.0	6.4
Not tied	3.0	4.5
Unrestrained		
In chair	34.9	20.1
Ambulatory	35.2	13.4

Note: $p < .01$.

once. The reports from staff incorporated one week of usual care. The two methods of assessing the use of restraints led to consistent findings that residents on comparison units were more often physically restrained.

PREDICTING THE USE OF RESTRAINTS THROUGH OBSERVATIONAL DATA

As with the use of medications, we next studied the influence of multiple variables on restraint use. Fourteen independent variables (potential confounders), which were postulated to contribute to physical restraint use, were included in the model. These included six facility characteristics: the state in which the facility was located, status as a dementia or comparison unit, staffing patterns, facility size, ownership status, and percentage of residents in the facility on medicaid. It also included eight resident characteristics: age, ADL status, past history of hip fracture, a past history of other fractures, frequency of family visits, mental status (as noted in the MOSES), behavioral problems (as noted in the MOSES), and physical abusiveness (as noted in the MOSES). An interaction term involved the type of setting and the state, exploring the differences among units in the five different states. Using logistic regression, a statistical technique, all the above variables were studied. A $p = .05$ criterion was used for inclusion in the final model.

Even in the model that included all potential predictors and simultaneously adjusted or controlled for all their possible effects, we found residents on the comparison units more likely to be restrained. Our final model identified five significant predictors. These were ADL status, mental status, staffing patterns, state, and unit status.

The more severe the ADL impairment, the greater the use of physical restraints. Unit status was also highly predictive, with the odds of restraint use in residents of comparison units approximately five times that of dementia units. In addition, residents in the moderate and high mental status impairment categories were nearly three times as likely to be restrained when compared with residents having low mental status impairment. A staffing pattern of 27 to 30 nursing hours per week per resident was associated with somewhat elevated odds of restraint use. Finally, residents of Ohio were more likely to be restrained than residents of the other four states.

We conclude that demented residents receiving traditional care are more often physically restrained than those in dementia units. This is the case even when we controlled for other variables that may have explained frequent use of restraints. It seemed that the dementia units resorted to other techniques for managing disruptive behavior or for ensuring resident safety, the main reasons cited for restraining a person. It may be that the total environment or milieu of a dementia unit promotes the philosophy that a resident should not be physically restrained.

THE USE OF CHEMICAL RESTRAINTS

For purposes of this analysis, a resident was considered chemically restrained if given a major tranquilizer such as haloperidol (Haldol), a minor tranquilizer such as diazepam (Valium), a hypnotic such as triazolam (Halcion), or a combination drug that included a major or minor tranquilizer on a routine basis. All other residents, including those on antidepressant agents such as amitriptyline (Elavil) alone, were not considered chemically restrained. Information on routinely administered drugs was collected through the review of medical records during the site visits.

A total of 54.7 percent of dementia unit residents were not taking any form of chemical restraint; however, 45.3 percent were receiving one or more of these drugs. On the comparison units, 56.6 percent of residents were not taking any form of these drugs, as opposed to 43.4 percent who were receiving these medications. These findings are listed in table 2.13. There were no statistically significant differences in the two settings (chi-square with 1 degree of freedom = 0.22, $p = .64$). That is, residents on the dementia units were chemically restrained no less than residents on comparison units. This finding was in contrast to that regarding physical restraints, both reported and observed, where a difference in the two settings was apparent.

TABLE 2.13   Use of Chemical Restraints (%)

	Dementia Unit Residents (N = 307)	Comparison Unit Residents (N = 318)
Chemically restrained	45.3	43.4
Not chemically restrained	54.7	56.6

Note: $p = .64$.

PREDICTING THE USE OF CHEMICAL RESTRAINTS

Next we studied the influence of certain variables on chemical restraint use, again using the statistical method multivariate logistic regression. The same fourteen independent variables were included in our model as had been used to study physical restraint use.

Physically abusive behavior was a significant predictor of chemical restraint use. The odds of chemical restraint use are roughly twice as great for a resident who has hit or shoved another resident or a staff member during the past week than for a resident who has not hit or shoved anyone. Other significant predictors were: age (the odds of receiving such medication is about one-half as great for those over 85 years of age as for residents under 75 years of age); family visitation (the odds of being chemically restrained were more than one and a half times greater among residents who had family visitors more than once a week, compared with those having visitors less frequently; and severe impairment of mental status. In addition, large facilities tended to use chemical restraints at lower rates; among residents in facilities having more than two hundred residents, the odds of being chemically restrained were about two-thirds of those found in smaller facilities. These results simultaneously controlled for the effects of all predictive variables. Status as a dementia unit or comparison unit was included in this predictive model because of its role in sample selection; it was not a significant predictor of chemical restraint use.

We conclude that while the residents of dementia units are less physically restrained than residents receiving traditional care, the use of chemical restraints was similar in both settings.

References

Burnside, I. (ed.). 1984. *Working with the elderly: Group Process and Techniques*, 2nd ed. Monterey, Calif: Wadsworth Health Sciences Division.

Coons, D. H., and Weaverdyck, S. E. 1986. Wesley Hall: A residential unit for persons with Alzheimer's disease and related disorders. In Taira, E. (ed.), *Therapeutic Interventions for the Person with Dementia*. New York: Haworth.

LeSage, J. 1982. Drug therapy in long-term facilities. *Nursing Clinics of North America* 17: 331–40.

Mace, N. L., and Rabins, P. V. 1981. *The 36-Hour Day: A Family Guide to Caring for Persons with Alzheimer's Disease, Related Dementing Illnesses, and Memory Loss in Later Life*. Baltimore: Johns Hopkins University Press.

McArthur, M. G. 1988. Exercise therapy for the Alzheimer's patient and caregiver. *American Journal of Alzheimer's Care and Related Disorders and Research* 3: 36–39.

Weiner, A. S. 1987. A nationwide survey of special units. In Kalicki, A. C. (ed.), *Confronting Alzheimer's Disease*. Owings Mills, Md.: Rynd Communications.

3

A Descriptive Typology
of Dementia Units

DEBORAH T. GOLD

With the knowledge that the number and proportion of demented older adults needing institutional care are growing quickly and that high-quality dementia care settings are difficult to find, this chapter has two major goals. First, the qualities of acceptable long-term care settings for dementia patients are identified briefly. Second, a typological structure for categorizing dementia care settings is described in detail. Hopefully, this typology will provide guidelines for those looking for high-quality institutional care for demented patients.

At this point, empirical evidence to show that dementia units provide more effective care than that provided in other settings is not available. But for the purposes of this discussion, we assume that the specific therapeutic care in a dementia unit is a unique care modality different from routine care in other settings. Therefore, the categorization explained below includes only dementia units.

Methods

From 31 dementia units systematically studied (see introduction and Appendix for study methods), subjective site visit notes were available on

28 units in the five states studied. The data gathered for the evaluation of the settings themselves were narratives. These subjective perceptions focused on the quality of care or, more broadly, the quality of life possible within each institution. Characteristics mentioned in the narratives include decor, external environment (i.e., neighborhood in which the home was located), physical layout of the units in which memory-impaired residents lived, the existence and use of a day-room or activities room, the apparent commitment of the staff and administration, and the observed interaction among staff and residents. These descriptions of the care settings were transcribed verbatim so that all data could be used effectively in the identification of high- or low-quality care.

The question of the reliability of these data must be raised here. Three different evaluators visited these nursing homes: a physician, a nurse, and a research assistant. Although site visits were made jointly by these data collectors to several facilities, in no instance were subjective notes compiled by more than one individual for a given facility. Therefore, the reliability of individual observations cannot be determined. Another problem exists in that no predetermined list of characteristics to be evaluated was developed before the observations were made. Thus, each evaluator emphasized certain characteristics (e.g., decor or resident privacy) that differed from those emphasized by the other investigators.

The verbatim transcripts were analyzed by three independent raters (different from the evaluators) using the constant comparative analytic method (Glazer and Strauss 1967, Gold 1989). A subsample of the primary analytic variables and their rating values is found in table 3.1.

As table 3.1 illustrates, a multidimensional perspective was used to assess the quality of care in these environments. The variables can be loosely divided into four aspects: physical facility, resident behaviors and activities, quality of staff, and quality of administration. A high-quality long-term care facility must excel in all of these dimensions. Problems in one aspect of a dementia unit inevitably lead to problems in the others because of the interactive nature of the care setting. However, for purposes of evaluation, we have attempted to tease out the differences both within and among these four dimensions.

After all transcripts had been reviewed, the patterns of ratings in various dimensions were compared. This comparison allowed transcripts to be grouped into categories that show meaningful similarities and differences. Using the categories developed by this constant comparative method, we constructed a typology that contains general guidelines for categorizing care settings for memory-impaired older people. Specific typological categories are described below.

TABLE 3.1   Key Variables Used in the Development of a Typology of Care Settings for Cognitively Impaired Older Adults

Variable	Coding Categories
Community environment	0 = unfavorable, 1 = favorable
External appearance	0 = bad, 1 = good
Public area appearance	0 = bad, 1 = good
Maintenance	0 = poor, 1 = good
Cleanliness	0 = dirty, 1 = clean
Unit layout	0 = poor, 1 = good
Decoration	0 = institutional, 1 = homey
Noise level	0 = noisy, 1 = quiet
Malodorousness	0 = yes, 1 = no
Inside ambiance	0 = depressing, 1 = cheerful
Resident population size	0 = large, 1 = small
Facility size for resident population	0 = crowded, 1 = uncrowded
Resident	
Room facilities	0 = shared, 1 = private
Appearance	0 = poor, 1 = well-groomed
Ambulation	0 = bedridden, 1 = ambulatory
Functional status	0 = low, 1 = moderate to high
Behavioral problems	0 = yes, 1 = no
Restraints (physical or chemical)	0 = yes, 1 = no
Location	0 = rooms, 1 = common areas
Activity level	0 = low, 1 = high
Wandering	0 = yes, 1 = no
Between-resident interaction	0 = low, 1 = high
Staff	
Attitude toward residents	0 = apathetic, 1 = caring
Stress level	0 = high, 1 = low
Responsiveness	0 = poor, 1 = responsive
Involvement	0 = uninvolved, 1 = involved
Activities director	0 = no, 1 = yes
Administration	
Philosophy	0 = maintenance, 1 = therapeutic
Criteria	0 = lax, 1 = strict
Attitude toward residents	0 = indifferent, 1 = involved
Involvement in resident care	0 = no, 1 = yes

THE TYPOLOGY

Six distinct care-setting types emerged from our analyses. Each type has unique characteristics so that it can stand alone, yet all types have the same underlying theme. This typology is not arranged in a strictly hierarchical order; it cannot be interpreted as based on an interval scale. Instead, each type represents a unique category that may be distinct from other categories for reasons other than a unidimensional "better-worse" comparison. For example, if one type of dementia unit takes only residents who still have substantial cognitive ability, is that better or worse than another type which takes dementia residents regardless of the level of disease severity? Such judgments cannot be made along a positive or negative continuum. And although some categories may seem qualitatively better than others, it is more appropriate to view typological divisions as different rather than better or worse. The typology of care settings is described below, and combinations of characteristics that led to the conceptual and pragmatic distinctions between them are highlighted.

The first type of dementia unit is called the *Ideal*. Any unit assigned to this category is supervised by an administration that is knowledgeable about dementia and various care options. These units have a therapeutic rather than a maintenance philosophy of care. More specifically, these units provide activities and other sources of cognitive and interpersonal stimulation rather than simply acting as boarding houses that provide shelter and meals. The administrators and trained professionals in the Ideal unit are experienced at providing care for memory-impaired residents. They express genuine concern for staff and residents alike. Furthermore, the administration cooperates in multiple areas with each care unit so that maximally effective humane care is provided.

The Ideal dementia unit is located in favorable external surroundings—that is, in a middle-class or better neighborhood that is safe and well maintained. The care setting itself is pristine; cleanliness is a major goal of the Ideal unit. Those who enter the Ideal setting are aware of its crisp, bright, and cheerful atmosphere. All public and common areas have a homey atmosphere, and attempts to personalize the surroundings for each resident are evident. Individual residents have a great deal of privacy (i.e., private rooms and baths), and each private room is decorated with the resident's personal possessions.

Residents are not permitted to languish in bed or remain uninvolved with continuing activities. In fact, an activities director is constantly busy, leading a variety of different activities all the time, and the staff in general makes a genuine effort to get residents out of bed, groomed, and into public areas. Residents found in Ideal settings are typically clean, ambulatory, well behaved, cooperative, and cheerful. Their functional levels are quite high, and their cognitive impairments relatively mild. Thus, directors of Ideal units do not incur some of the care burdens of residents with severe cognitive impairments. Further, most of the residents are middle or upper class and pay privately rather than through Medicaid.

Staff-resident interactions are pleasant and positive in the Ideal setting. All levels of staff are well trained and have learned the specialty care appropriate for dementia residents. The adequacy of the staff-resident ratio keeps staff stress at unusually low levels. Each staff member has thorough knowledge about all residents on the unit; each staff member is efficient and contributes greatly to the smooth running of the unit.

The majority of Ideal dementia units are run by professionals who believe that dementia residents should be segregated from persons whose impairments are not related to dementia. Only in this way can activities and services be directed toward the overarching needs of memory-impaired residents.

The Ideal unit inspires confidence and comfort in the relatives of the residents. No one who understood the needs of dementia residents and was looking for a permanent long-term care setting would hesitate to place a patient in a facility with these benefits.

The second type of dementia unit resembles the Ideal type quite closely. The *Uncultivated* dementia unit is located in a facility in a safe and well-maintained neighborhood. Emphasis is placed on building and unit cleanliness and maintenance. There is not the consistent freshly scrubbed look of the Ideal unit, but without doubt the professionals involved here concern themselves with the outside appearance of the unit. The staff are extremely attentive to the residents and have as one major goal each resident's personal hygiene. The "nursing home stench" that we associate with a long-term care setting is absent. Residents here have private or semiprivate rooms and baths. All areas, including public ones, are decorated in a pleasant and cheerful way. Once again, an observer would see personal objects in the resident's rooms. As was true in the Ideal setting, residents in the Uncultivated settings have relatively mild dementia and thus are ambulatory. They can involve themselves in group activities and establish close relationships with staff members.

The highly trained staff found in most Uncultivated units should be able to provide a level of resident care that is quite good. Staff-resident interactions are positive for the most part, but the staff size is sometimes not sufficient to meet the constant demands of all the residents. As a result, stress for staff in this dementia unit can be quite high. Unlike the Ideal unit, staff members in the Uncultivated unit can be faced with administrators who, though they are supportive, exacerbate the frustrations of trying to care for too many residents with too few professionals.

It is clear that the primary difference between an Ideal and an Uncultivated unit is at the administrative level. Instead of involved and knowledgeable people to direct the overall administration of the dementia unit, Uncultivated settings have directors who lack dementia-specific training, have little experience in working with any long-term care population, and often appear primarily concerned with monitoring working hours and keeping costs down. Staff members in the Uncultivated unit are not specifically assigned by level of skill (i.e., those with the most complete dementia care training may not be caregivers of dementia residents); thus, they are less efficacious than might be expected. The relatively high stress level and a high resident–staff ratio inevitably leads to superficial knowledge about each resident and little individual attention.

With a bit of administrative awareness and nurturing, these Uncultivated units could be turned into Ideal ones. Hiring enough staff to handle the resident load, carefully monitoring staffing placements, encouraging collaboration among disciplines, and providing effective staff training are the major tasks the administration needs to undertake. The differences between these two types of care settings affect resident care both directly and indirectly; however, the source of problems is not at the resident-care level. And because of the high quality of every other aspect of these homes, the Uncultivated units could be converted to *Ideal* care settings with a little effort and at low cost.

The next two types of dementia units are reminiscent of the old adage, "Don't judge a book by its cover." In both cases, the quality of the external surroundings is misleading. First, the *Heart of Gold* unit usually has a less than appealing appearance. The buildings are old and dilapidated; little of the available budget is "wasted" on external maintenance. The neighborhoods in which these units are located frequently are some of the worst in a city. When visitors or residents walk inside, they are greeted with dim lighting, shiny and slippery floors, and a poorly designed unit layout. The quasi-institutional appearance precludes the presence of many personal items or homey furniture. This type of home is generally nonprofit rather than proprietary, and it might be assumed that the staff here had a maintenance rather than a therapeutic care philosophy. In contrast to units that discharge residents with advanced dementia, the Heart of Gold unit tends to contain a wider functional spectrum of residents, and its resident mix becomes more impaired as the unit ages.

Yet if visitors can ignore the building's facade, they will see a staff that is friendly and responsive to resident needs. The inside appearance is antithetical to that outside. Cleanliness is evident, with no unpleasant odor. Residents are out of their rooms, either in geri-chairs or in a dayroom. The overall level of resident functioning is considerably lower than that at either the Ideal or the Uncultivated setting. Many residents are simply too impaired to participate in the arranged activities, but one-to-one contact is frequent and therapeutic. Thus, residents with dementia receive the same attention as others with less severe cognitive impairments. An observer would note an unusually high level of contact between staff and residents, much of it initiated by staff members. The resident–staff ratio is not ideal, but it is low enough so that staff members experience only mild stress—largely when substitutes for absent members cannot be found. Heart of Gold settings are rare, but it is important to note that the residents in these units receive high-quality physical and psychosocial care.

It would take a significant investment to upgrade this care setting. Problems with dim lighting, poor layout, and other structural issues could, however, be overcome with sufficient financial backing. The major negative variable that cannot be modified is the location of the home in which this unit is found. The Heart of Gold care setting often results from a changing neighborhood. Potential residents or family members typically bypass this location on the basis of appearance alone. Ignoring these units is a shame, for the quality of care provided is far better than that provided in some of the more externally attractive institutions.

Unfortunately, the antithesis of the Heart of Gold unit also exists. This is called *Rotten at the Core*. Dementia units of this type are newer and well maintained. Typically, they are located in well-established neighborhoods, and the buildings and grounds are well manicured. Upon entering an institutional setting that includes a Rotten at the Core unit, people are aware that a large investment has been made in external appearances. The lighting is excellent, the floors are clean but not slippery, the furniture is homey and comfortable, and all public areas are meticulously organized. The technical level of nursing care in these settings is quite high, with residents receiving medicines and other routine nursing services at appropriate times. If bright lights and cheerful halls, private rooms, and homey furniture alone could provide quality care to memory-impaired residents, the Rotten at the Core unit would receive high marks. However, when the facade is penetrated and the real kind of care given in these units is revealed, we find that the Rotten at the Core unit consists of a staff and administration that provide (1) maintenance rather than therapy, (2) technically correct care without warmth, empathy, or affection, and (3) apathetic, sometimes overtly unfriendly service. Residents interact with staff very infrequently, by staff choice. Those residents who have lived in a Rotten at the Core unit for any length of time frequently develop a flat affect, quite possibly as a result of minimal human interaction.

Most resources in this care setting are put toward environmental improvements, little toward resident needs. Unlike the caring staff seen at the Heart of Gold units, Rotten at the Core staff rarely initiate touching or conversation. Residents remain in their rooms with no programmed activities. This, as might be expected, leads to low staff stress. Externally, this setting appears to be perfect. Only closer examination reveals that it is Rotten at the Core. The existence of this type of unit should teach consumers to be especially careful to analyze both the appearance of the care setting and the quality of care provided there.

The fifth type of unit for cognitively impaired residents is called the *Institutional* unit. This type has a positive external environment, and the structure itself is well-maintained if a bit traditional. Inside, the Institutional setting is clean and quiet, much like the corridors of an acute-care wing of a hospital. In fact, this setting resembles a hospital in more than just appearance and general atmosphere. The decor is uniform but lacks the homey touches or residents' personal decorations that make the Ideal or Uncultivated settings comfortable and comforting. Residents live in both private and semiprivate rooms, yet no evidence of their individuality is seen anywhere. Floors are uncarpeted but are kept clean. The overall atmosphere exudes passivity with the uniform and traditional health care ambiance.

Residents here receive first-rate physical care; they are well groomed, neat, and cooperative. Many, if not most, of the residents have other serious (comorbid) conditions or advanced immobility that precludes their getting out of bed and participating in organized activities. Continuous bed rest leads to both physical and cognitive debilitation. Little interaction occurs among the residents themselves, in part because those in Institutional settings are typically far more impaired than those in some of the previously described settings. Also, because their physical condition is also quite poor, residents on the Institutional unit need skilled nursing care much of the time.

Those needs are almost a perfect fit with the philosophy of administrators of Institutional dementia units. These administrators focus on maintenance and monitoring, with no therapeutic dimension. If the unit has an activity program for dementia residents, it is extremely limited. The starched and organized atmosphere of such a care unit mandates that it be well run with low staff stress and a low resident–staff ratio. Staff members who accept work in such a setting are typically efficient and responsive, have deep rather than superficial knowledge of the residents, and express caring and support in a sincere way. What they do not (or cannot) do is provide stimulation and interaction with and among the residents. For cognitively impaired residents who need highly skilled nursing care (especially those in the final stages of dementia), the Institutional setting coincides almost perfectly with their needs.

The sixth type of dementia unit, the *Limited*, inspires confidence and hopefulness at first glance. Limited units appear well run and well maintained. They are typically found in acceptable neighborhoods. While the building and grounds are not manicured, they are kept neat. The internal environment has some shortcomings when compared to the Ideal or

Uncultivated units, but these shortcomings are hard to specify. Floors are clean but not sparkling. The furniture is homey and comfortable, but there is either too little or too much of it. The rooms are typically semiprivate with shared baths, but quarters are often overcrowded because of administrative reluctance to turn potential residents (and profit) away. The odor of feces and urine, while slight, is ever present.

In the Limited care setting (unlike the Uncultivated), problems do not reside in the hands of a poor administration. Limited units usually have administrators with a solid base of experience and knowledge about ways in which to meet residents' needs. The shortcomings here are found primarily in the staff. Interaction with residents does not occur on a large or frequent scale. The lack of programmed activities for dementia residents is obvious. The few physical impediments mentioned above (e.g., crowding, too little or too much furniture, malodorousness) are eminently correctable, but no attempts are made to improve the situation. These limitations stand in the way of providing optimal care to the resident. Over the long term, residents with cognitive impairments may worsen more quickly in a Limited setting than in another setting with well-planned activities and a caring and involved staff.

Although the Limited unit gives the impression of being well run, efficient, and beneficial, the general premise is that, with additional effort and specialized care for dementia residents along several critical dimensions, this unit could move into the Ideal category. The impediments of these improvements lie in the hands of the staff. Only an administrator with a strong will and good interpersonal style will be able to convince the staff that resident interactions must improve. The raw material for outstanding care is present in the Limited unit; it just hasn't been used to its fullest potential.

Unacceptable Care Settings: How Can We Know?

In describing the above types of dementia units, a wide variety has been introduced. The units range from almost perfect to indifferent and uncaring. In the sample of dementia units used for this study, none functioned so badly that it deserved to be classified completely negatively. In part, this is unfortunate, because there are surely some dementia units in this country where care is egregious, staff interactions are prescribed and without affect, and no sense of caring exists. Below are some of the negative qualities that might be visible in the least desirable dementia units.

An unacceptable dementia unit would have evolved into a prototype for lackadaisical nursing home care. Negative sensory input from the combination of feces, urine, and cleaning solutions and from harsh and noisy sounds throughout the unit would overwhelm the casual observer. In settings that are least care oriented often reside the most cognitively impaired and physically debilitated residents. They either remain in bed all day nearly comatose, wander aimlessly through the halls, or slouch restrained and mute in a line of chairs facing the nursing station. Under these circumstances, no activities would be provided for cognitively impaired residents. The daily challenge is to control them and to avoid self-harm. These units might appear clean, especially around holidays when families are likely to visit, but on the whole no one would seem concerned about the dust and dirt gathering in residents' rooms or the common areas.

Some interaction between staff and residents might occur in this setting, but its nature would be instrumental rather than affective. The use of physical and chemical restraints would increase as the days progressed because behaviorally problematic residents would not be tolerated. Staff members and administrators would appear to live for the hours they spend away from these units on weekends, holidays, or vacations. The hours "in house" would be borne not with stoicism but with complaints and without much effort.

Often, the primary goal of units that offer substandard care is maximum monetary gain with minimum staff effort. Under these conditions, administrators would consistently look for ways to cut costs and raise income. Thus, any attempts to improve the appearance of the unit would be halfhearted. The only concerted effort would be a "chart buffing" and resident cleanup in anticipation of a site visit from a regulatory or certifying agency. Clearly, this would be a care setting in which administration and staff needs would receive top priority. The results would be insensitivity to patient comfort, lack of maintenance, and a self-serving commitment from staff and administration. These goals would effectively reduce quality of care to nothing.

One tragic dimension of the residents in such a unit is that they would likely not have families to watch out for them or act as advocates. Their weakness and debilitation would keep them in bed, and the lack of interaction might make them more vulnerable to the negative consequences of their dementia.

These ineffective and inhumane care settings would provide only resident maintenance rather than any therapeutic care. Such a stance on a dementia unit would be antithetical to a dementia unit's stated purpose. But some units might slide into a morass of conflicts between administration, staff, and residents. In such units, it might be expected that behavioral problems would run rampant and lead to high staff stress. Chemical and physical restraints would appear to be the only means by which the staff could control wandering or abusive residents.

Lax admissions criteria would mean that these units would fill with residents inappropriate for a dementia unit. Rather than screen out people with serious physical comorbidity or mental disorders such as alcoholism, schizophrenia, or mental retardation, directors of ineffective units might encourage the recruitment of any patients. An empty bed means a day without third-party reimbursement. Each day during which a bed is full means a day for which the unit is reimbursed by insurance, primarily Medicaid.

Conclusions

No resident with progressive dementia should have to live in a care setting as poor as the hypothetical dementia unit just described. Fortunately, care settings of this type are becoming less evident and appear particularly unlikely to appear when administrative and staff effort go into the development of a dementia unit.

Regardless, family members must be diligent about any nursing home placement. A distraught adult child might easily be fooled into ignoring a Heart of Gold unit in favor of one that is Rotten at the Core. Superficial appearances can lead us to conclude incorrectly that a care setting is of the highest, or lowest, quality. Thus, superficial approaches to care selection should be replaced with a thorough examination of any care setting. Furthermore, recommendations from other residents or their families are more likely to be true than are public relations brochures or pep talks from nursing home directors.

One primary factor that reveals quality of care in a dementia unit is the amount and kind of staff-resident interaction. Staff should not be so busy that they cannot interact informally with residents during the day. Staff should initiate some contact with residents beyond bringing their meals or cleaning them up. If most of this interaction is based on nursing procedure or triggered by "emergencies" (i.e., incontinence, falls), the staff may be genuinely disinterested in the quality of care they provide. An apathetic staff can prove to be one of the major barriers to good care.

A second factor that should play a role in long-term decisions for demented older adults is the level of training in special dementia care among the staff and administration. If a unit provides activities and interactions that are the same as those in most nursing homes and if chemical and physical restraint is frequent, it is most likely that maintenance of residents is the primary goal. On the other hand, if activities are available and appropriate and control becomes a means to an end rather than the end itself, the administration and staff most likely believe in a therapeutic approach to dementia management. Some demented residents cannot benefit from the therapeutic approach, but for those that can, it is critical to find a unit on which this kind of care occurs.

The typology presented in this chapter must be interpreted with caution; the delineation of categories is still preliminary. The typology is designed to paint a broad picture of the various kinds of dementia units, providing families and researchers the background necessary for understanding the broad spectrum of care provided. It is critical to realize that the categories discussed here are based on a combination of data from various nursing homes. No single home matches any of the categories perfectly. But any dementia unit should have enough characteristics in common with one of the types to allow some pairing. This will give observers a broadbrush understanding of what may go on inside a care setting.

The consumer must evaluate the potential, as well as the actual, quality of any long-term care setting. Some are so poorly administered that a mere glance from outside provides convincing negative evidence and no suggestion of any forthcoming change. Others take great care to mislead potential clients; the facility's staff sweeps the "dirt" under the rugs during visiting hours or at the prospect of a new client. In still other cases, it becomes obvious that only minor adjustments in resident care or administrative attitudes would be necessary to move a nursing home unit from one category to another. The typology can also serve to warn potential clients about the hidden side of institutional care in dementia units.

The responsibility for quality long-term care is shared by multiple groups of interested people. Part of it lies with the government, especially in terms of economic issues. But some of the responsibility lies in the hands of the general public and, more specifically, in the hands of family members of demented older adults. The development of this typology to help family members sift the wheat from the chaff of long-term care facilities is only the first in a series of steps essential to maintain or improve the quality of care in dementia units. All interested parties must work together to demand sufficient openings in high-quality settings such as dementia units so that those who suffer from Alzheimer's and related dementias can live out their lives under the best possible conditions.

References

Glaser, B. G., and Strauss, A. L. 1967. *The Discovery of Grounded Theory: Strategies for Qualitative Research*. Chicago: Aldine.

Gold, D. T. 1989. Sibling relations in old age: A typology. *International Journal of Aging and Human Development* 28: 37–51.

II

Characteristics of Residents with Dementia

4

Characteristics of Residents with Dementia

PHILIP D. SLOANE AND LAURA J. MATHEW

Good nursing home care for people with Alzheimer's disease and related disorders requires that providers have an understanding of the characteristics and needs of those afflicted. Our study gathered detailed information on 625 dementia residents in 63 nursing homes. This represents a data base from which much can be learned about nursing home residents with dementia. This chapter describes the 625 dementia residents we studied, and through them, what we learned in general about nursing home residents with dementia. It contrasts residents in dementia units with those in comparison facilities who have similar diagnoses. It also describes similarities and differences between for-profit (proprietary) and nonprofit facilities.

For additional comparison, we cite data from the 1985 National Nursing Home Survey (NNHS), which we obtained on tape from the National Center for Health Statistics. The NNHS identified dementia residents on the basis of responses to the question: "According to (the resident)'s medical record does he/she currently have . . . senile dementia/chronic and organic brain syndrome?" With respect to comparative data from the NNHS, the reader should keep in mind that the methods of that survey are not identical to ours. We have attempted to compare similar items and categories, and in some cases we have used identical questions. In many cases, however, the wording or category structure of questions differed somewhat between our survey and the NNHS's.

Demographic Characteristics and Background Health Status of Current Residents

Data obtained from medical records of 307 residents of dementia units and 318 residents of comparison units were used to compare basic demographic features and diagnoses. Our analyses revealed clear differences between the two sets of residents: The dementia unit group was younger, almost entirely white, and more frequently married to a living spouse. Dementia units contained a lower proportion of female residents (though they still predominated). Length of stay in nursing homes was shorter for dementia unit residents than for the comparison group. Also, a specific diagnosis of Alzheimer's disease was more common among dementia unit residents. Little difference was noted, however, in the prevalence of selected morbid conditions between the two groups.

AGE, RACE, SEX, AND MARITAL STATUS

On average, residents of dementia units were about three years younger than residents of comparison units. The mean ages of dementia unit residents (80.0 years) and comparison unit residents (83.2 years) were significantly different when tested statistically ($p < .001$). Dementia unit residents were more likely to be white (94.46 versus 86.79 percent); these results were also statistically significant ($p = .011$). Specialized unit residents were more likely to be male than comparison unit residents ($p = .029$). They were also more likely to be married to a living spouse ($p = .007$). These results are summarized in table 4.1.

DEMENTIA DIAGNOSES

The majority of dementia unit residents (58 percent) had a specific diagnosis of Alzheimer's disease listed on the medical record. This contrasted with our comparison units, where the majority (75 percent) had a nonspecific dementia diagnosis, such as organic brain syndrome, senility, or chronic confusion. These differences were highly significant statistically ($p < .001$). Other dementias appearing on medical records, such as the cerebrovascular dementias (cerebral arteriosclerosis, multi-infarct dementia, and Binswanger's disease) and specific organic brain diagnosis (such as Pick's disease, parkinsonism with dementia, alcoholic brain disease, and Huntington's disease) did not differ significantly between our dementia unit and comparison groups. These results are summarized in table 4.2.

TABLE 4.1   Residents' Demographic Characteristics and Length of Stay

	Current Residents		Discharged Residents	
	Dementia Units (N = 306)	Comparison Units (N = 318)	Dementia Units (N = 152)	Comparison Units (N = 149)
Mean age (yr)	80.0	83.2	80.1	83.9
Race (%)				
White	94.5	86.8	96.0	87.0
Black	3.6	8.8	2.7	9.4
Hispanic	2.0	4.1	1.3	3.6
Other	0.0	0.3	0.0	0.0
Sex (%)				
Female	74.9	82.1	71.0	82.6
Male	25.1	17.9	29.0	17.4
Married to living spouse (%)	23.9	15.3	—	—
Time since admission (%)				
<3 mo	13.6	8.8	33.1	32.0
3–12 mo	14.6	24.6	25.8	20.7
1–3 yr	38.4	40.4	29.1	21.3
>3 yr	33.4	26.2	11.9	26.0

TABLE 4.2   Dementia Diagnoses of Study Subjects

Diagnosis	In Dementia Units (N = 307)	In Comparison Units (N = 318)	Chi-square	p
Alzheimer's disease	57.6%	23.6%	73.9	<.001
Cerebrovascular dementia	6.8	8.5	.4	n.s.
Other specific organic brain disease with dementia	2.6	2.2	.0	n.s.
Nonspecific dementia	39.1	74.5	78.7	<.001

Note: Totals exceed 100% because some subjects had more than one dementia diagnosis; n.s., not significant.

Interpretation of this diagnostic information is rendered difficult by the lack of diagnostic standards and resulting inconsistencies in terminology. There appears to be a trend to use the term Alzheimer's disease where in the past a more nonspecific label was applied, and dementia units seem to be at the forefront of this trend. From informal conversations with physicians we met during the study, nonspecific diagnoses tended to be preferred by two groups: (1) well-informed but cautious physicians who hesitated to make an Alzheimer's diagnosis because the only truly confirmatory test is a brain biopsy; and (2) physicians who are relatively unfamiliar with recent developments in geriatric medicine (i.e., the redefinition of Alzheimer's as the most prevalent diagnosis in the elderly demented and delineation of clinical criteria for vascular dementias) and apply diagnostic labels they learned decades ago. We are uncertain, however, that any meaningful difference in the clinical picture of presentation exists between the average "Alzheimer's" resident in a nursing home and the average "organic brain syndrome" (O.B.S.) resident in another facility. As we show later, the degree of mental status and behavioral impairments in the dementia unit and comparison groups was similar.

THE PREVALENCE OF COMORBID CONDITIONS

The presence of other diseases (comorbid conditions) in residents with Alzheimer's disease or other dementias can lead to additional disability. This comorbidity often resu s in additional medical and nursing care needs. Because of this, we documented the extent to which comorbidities existed among our dementia unit and comparison samples. We did this by recording up to five additional diagnoses found in the records of our study sample.

In identifying these diagnoses, we reviewed the admission face sheet, which often contained reasons for the previous hospitalization and failed to reflect current problems; the nursing problem lists; and the physicians' annual physical examination results. No more than six diagnoses, including the dementia diagnosis, were recorded. In some cases, more than six diagnoses were listed in residents' records. Thus, while we attempted to list the six most important diagnoses for the resident, it is possible that our estimates of the prevalence of comorbid conditions are low. To aid comparison, we have computed similar measures for demented and nondemented nursing home residents using data tapes from the 1985 National Nursing Home Survey. The results are summarized in table 4.3.

Comparison of comorbidity rates between dementia units and comparison units reveals mixed results. The rates of cardiac and cardiovascular diagnoses were similar. The fact that fewer dementia unit residents

TABLE 4.3 Prevalence of Selected Comorbid Conditions, with Comparison Data from the National Nursing Home Survey

Diagnosis	In Dementia Units (N = 307)	In Comparison Units (N = 318)	Chi-square	p	1985 NNHS Data Dementia	1985 NNHS Data Nondementia
Cardiac disease	31.3%	37.7%	2.89	n.s.	37.5%	34.9%
Currently using cardiovascular medication	42.7	55.0	9.55	.05	n.a.	n.a.
History of stroke	5.2	11.0	7.00	<.01	7.0	10.2
History of fracture						
Hip	9.8	15.7	4.96	<.05	3.9	5.4
Other site	1.6	4.7	4.81	<.05	n.a.	n.a.
Visual impairment	12.4	9.4	1.40	n.s.	n.a.	n.a.
Deafness	2.3	2.8	0.19	n.s.	1.7	2.2

Note: n.s., not significant; n.a., not applicable.

were taking cardiovascular medications, however, may indicate that they had less severe disease. Significantly fewer dementia unit residents had a history of stroke, hip fracture, or other fracture. However, no significant differences were noted between the two groups in the prevalence of visual impairment or severe hearing less (deafness).

LENGTH OF STAY

We measured the length of stay (LOS) in two ways. LOS for this admission (LOS-A) was the length of time the resident had been continuously institutionalized in the same nursing home since admission or the last overnight hospitalization. LOS since first admitted for continuous nursing home care (LOS-NH) was determined by searching through the medical record, and in particular the social service notes, to determine when the individual last lived at home, a rest home, or some other less intensive level of care. The date of nursing home admission from home or after an intervening hospitalization was then used to determine LOS-NH. Because LOS-NH indicates how far back the average study subject was placed in a nursing home, it provides our best measure of the average duration of dementia among these subjects.

As measured by both LOS-A and LOS-NH, residents of dementia units have been institutionalized for a shorter time than comparison unit residents. The mean value of LOS-A was 587 days for dementia unit residents; for comparison unit residents it was 832 days. The difference between these means was highly significant statistically ($p < .001$). Table 4.1 shows the categorical distribution of LOS-A.

Overall length of stay in nursing homes differed even more. The mean value of LOS-NH was 821 days for the dementia unit group and 1,336 days for the comparison group, again a highly significant difference ($p < .001$). Thus, the average dementia unit resident had spent nearly a year and a half less in nursing homes than the average comparison unit resident. This suggests that dementia unit residents on average are earlier in their illness than comparison unit residents.

Recently Discharged Residents

A cross-sectional study underrepresents residents who do not stay long. These short-stay residents are usually defined as those who leave within three months of admission. They include people who are rehabilitated and return home, those in the last phases of terminal illness, those whose unstable health leads to rehospitalization, those who were inappropriately placed, and those who for behavioral or other reasons did not adjust to a nursing home. Such short-stay residents may comprise as many as half of admissions to nursing homes. Because their admissions are brief, however, they occupy only a small percentage of nursing home beds at any one time. Thus, they have less impact on daily operations of a nursing home than residents who remain longer. The characteristics of this group are important to understand, however, particularly in evaluating retention rates and planning admissions.

Such residents often differ from those who stay for long periods of time. To learn about them, we studied people with dementia diagnoses who had been discharged recently from the units we visited. Altogether, medical records of 152 recent discharges from dementia units and 149 recent discharges from comparison units were reviewed. Our findings are summarized in this section.

DEMOGRAPHIC CHARACTERISTICS AND LENGTH OF STAY

Our sample of discharged residents did not differ significantly from the current residents in terms of age, race, or sex (information on marital status was not obtained). Table 4.1 summarizes our findings. When we examined separately those residents who had been discharged within one month of admission, these similarities remained.

While we did not specifically document discharge rates, we observed during data collection that discharges were relatively infrequent in both the dementia and comparison units. Thus, turnover of demented residents seemed relatively slow in both settings. Based on this experience, we estimate that one discharge occurs per month for every 15 to 30 beds occupied by a dementia resident. Higher attrition rates exist in newly established units, since more of their residents are recent admissions. The likely explanation for the stability of these residents is that two of the most common reasons for rapid turnover of nursing home beds— rehabilitation and unstable medical status—are found less frequently in dementing illness.

REASONS FOR DISCHARGE

The final disposition of discharged residents differed considerably between dementia units and comparison units (see table 4.4). The specialized units seem to discharge residents to family and to other nursing homes at higher rates, whereas death and hospitalization are more common among comparison unit residents. This trend is most pronounced when we examine the figures for residents who stayed less than three months. Dementia units discharged 51 percent of short-term residents to their homes or to other nursing home situations, whereas comparison units discharged only 17 percent. The opposite relationship is present for death; 37 percent of short-stay residents in comparison units died, compared with only 10 percent in dementia units.

These data suggest that discharge policies of dementia units differ

TABLE 4.4   Final Disposition of Discharged Residents (%)

	All Discharged Residents		Those Discharged within 3 Months	
	Dementia Units (N = 149)	Comparison Units (N = 152)	Dementia Units (N = 47)	Comparison Units (N = 51)
Family	9.2	4.0	21.6	10.6
Another nursing home unit	27.0	8.1	29.4	6.4
Hospital	36.8	47.6	35.3	44.7
Funeral home	21.0	38.9	9.8	36.2
Other	5.9	1.3	3.9	2.1

from those of traditional nursing home units. As we discuss later in this book, many specialized units explicitly state that residents will be discharged when too impaired to benefit from some of the activities and behavioral interventions the unit offers. Data gathered on reasons for discharge support this conclusion: 10 percent of discharges from dementia units were because of "inappropriate placement," in contrast to only 1 percent of discharges from comparison units. The higher proportion of residents returning home from dementia units (table 4.4) may reflect either that rehabilitation occurs in certain cases, or that these units provide respite care.

Functional Status of Current Residents

Based on the literature on long-term care, discussions with nursing home staff, and our own experiences managing dementia residents, we believed that the dependency in activities of daily living (ADLs), communication problems, cognitive impairment, and behavioral problems were among the major determinants of care needs and of ability to participate in many programs. To describe residents consistently and to compare groups, we used standardized reporting instruments, which provide relatively reproducible measures of these factors.

The Multidimensional Observation Scale for Elderly Subjects (MOSES) questionnaire (Helmes et al. 1987) was the primary instrument used to study these factors. A 40-item questionnaire that must be completed by a staff member who knows the resident well, the MOSES covers five areas, each of which can be reported as a score: physical status (ADLs); mental status; mood (manifestations of anxiety or depression); overt behavioral problems; and socialization. Additional details about data collection using the MOSES are presented in the Appendix.

ACTIVITIES OF DAILY LIVING

Table 4.5 shows the basic ADL dependencies among dementia unit and comparison unit residents. In both settings, virtually all people with a dementia diagnosis need help bathing, grooming, and dressing. Most (69 percent in dementia units and 84 percent in comparison units) have some degree of incontinence. Problems with mobility and with transferring from a bed to a chair are also common.

Statistically significant differences between dementia unit and comparison unit residents were found in all ADLs studied. In each ADL, dementia unit residents were less dependent. The greatest differences were in mobility, transfer, toileting, and incontinence. Sixty percent of dementia unit residents could ambulate or wheel themselves independently, compared with 20 percent of comparison unit residents; 52 percent of dementia unit residents could transfer independently, compared with 21 percent of comparison unit residents; 38 percent of dementia residents required complete assistance with toileting, compared with 60 percent of comparison unit residents; and 44 percent of dementia unit residents were incontinent daily, compared with 61 percent of comparison unit residents.

Physical (ADL) Impairment Scale: Defining Levels of Dependency Using
MOSES *Scores*

We created a single variable, the physical impairment scale, to estimate relative disabilities of subjects in this sample. MOSES items 1 to 7 were used (dressing, bathing, grooming, toileting, mobility, transfer, and incontinence). The eighth ADL item in the MOSES, use of physical restraints, was omitted from our scale because we believe that it reflects policy more than it describes dependency. The seven items used are each scaled from 1 to 4, with 1 representing independence and 4, total dependence. A resident's score on the physical impairment scale was calculated by multiplying the mean score on the seven items by 100. We then used these scores to construct three categories of physical status: independent, intermediate, and totally dependent.

In the nursing home, "independence" is relative and usually implies independent mobility, toileting, and transfer, plus little or no incontinence. These "independent" residents often need supervision or some assistance with bathing, dressing, and grooming. On the basis of this definition and review of the MOSES instrument, we identified a total score of 140 on our seven ADL items as the upper limit for the independent group.

TABLE 4.5   Activities of Daily Living Status of Residents

Activity and Status	Dementia Unit Residents ($N = 307$)[a]	Comparison Unit Residents ($N = 318$)[a]	Chi-square (d.f. = 3)[b]	p
Dressing				
Independent	3.9%	6.6%	20.1	<.001
Minor supervision	15.0	7.9		
Frequent assistance	23.8	14.8		
Total care required	57.3	70.8		
Bathing				
Independent	0.6	1.3	13.6	.004
Minor supervision	6.2	6.3		
Frequent assistance	27.7	15.8		
Total care required	65.5	76.7		
Grooming				
Independent	2.3	4.8	15.6	.001
Minor supervision	13.0	8.9		
Frequent assistance	25.7	15.9		
Total care required	59.0	70.5		
Incontinence				
None	30.6	16.4	23.5	<.001
Night only	5.6	3.8		
Occasional	20.1	18.6		
> Once a day	43.8	61.2		
Toileting				
Independent	24.1	12.9	32.1	<.001
Minor supervision	13.0	8.5		
Frequent assistance	25.1	18.6		
Total care required	37.8	59.9		
Mobility				
Independent	60.5	19.5	124.8	<.001
Minor supervision	9.8	20.1		
Frequent assistance	16.0	17.0		
Total care required	13.7	43.4		
Transfer				
Independent	52.3	20.6	69.0	<.001
Minor supervision	2.3	1.9		
Frequent assistance	44.1	74.6		
Total care required	1.3	2.9		

[a] Actual numbers of subjects in the individual categories ranged between 304 and 307 for dementia unit residents, and between 312 and 318 for comparison unit residents. Some data are missing.
[b] d.f., degrees of freedom.

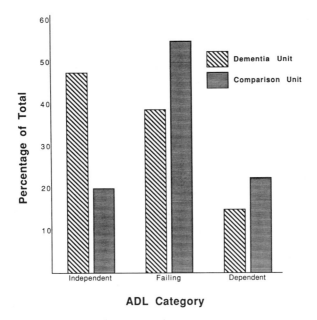

ADL Category

FIGURE 4.1 Activities of daily living (ADL): dementia units versus comparison units.

Because "totally dependent" people do not necessarily need to be completely bedridden, they might score 3 or 4 on transfer. A score of 3 on one other item was allowed, so that people who were completely dependent in all but one rated activity would still fall in the "totally dependent" group. Thus, we defined "totally dependent" people as those whose physical impairment score was 370 or greater.

Scores between 200 and 370 defined the "intermediate" group, those who are not completely dependent but are failing (require assistance) in continence or basic mobility parameters.

Comparison of ADL Dependency Scores between Dementia Units and Comparison Units

The overall mean ADL score for the 625 subjects in our study was 303. The mean score for dementia unit residents was 281; the mean score for comparison unit residents was 324. This difference was significant statistically ($p < .001$). The frequencies of residents found in the three categories (independent, intermediate or failing, and dependent) are displayed as figure 4.1; these categorical differences are also highly significant ($p < .001$).

In summary, these results document a high level of ADL dependency among dementia residents in the nursing home units we studied. Overall, nearly 50 percent of residents in the study were totally dependent. Another 30 percent were failing in one or more mobility measures or were incontinent. When dementia unit and control subjects are compared, it is apparent that functionally dependent subjects are concentrated in the comparison population. Dementia unit residents display a wider range of physical dependency and overall are less impaired.

COMMUNICATION SKILLS

The ability to communicate is measured by two items of the MOSES mental status scale: understanding communication, and verbal expression. Understanding communication (item 9) was rated on a four-point scale, with 1 representing clear understanding and 4 representing lack of any understanding. Verbal expression (item 10) was rated on a five-point scale, with 1 representing coherent, logical speech and 5 representing no spontaneous speech.

These two items were used to construct a continuous variable. The total score on the two questions was multiplied by 100, yielding an index that ranged from 200 to 900. Review of the distribution of this variable among our 625 subjects showed it to be relatively evenly distributed over the range of scores. Examination of cross-tabulations between the receptive and verbal communication scores showed a strong association. These characteristics supported the use of a combined score reported as a continuous variable. The use of a continuous variable to describe communication status made intuitive sense as well, because communication problems in dementia occur across a gradient, not falling into discrete categories but often progressing gradually over time.

Comparison of Communication Scores between Dementia Units and Comparison Units

As indicated by figure 4.2, the communication scores of dementia unit and comparison unit subjects covered virtually the entire available range (200 to 900). Thus, the communication skills of residents in both settings span a broad range, from understanding speech well and conversing fluently to neither understanding communication nor communicating verbally at all.

Little difference was noted in the reported communication abilities of residents in the two settings. The ability to understand communication was nearly identical in the dementia unit and comparison unit groups. There was a trend for dementia unit residents to be somewhat more verbal, but it did not reach statistical significance. These results are summarized in table 4.6.

Scores on the combined communication scale were similar between

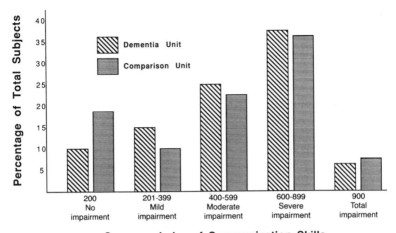

Score on Index of Communication Skills

FIGURE 4.2   Communication skills of residents: dementia units versus comparison units.

the samples. The mean score for dementia units was 516.0 and for comparison units, 518.6. The difference was not statistically significant (*t*-test with 621 degrees of freedom = .15, not significant).

MENTAL STATUS

Impaired mental status is probably the most distinctive feature of dementia. Whether the diagnosis is Alzheimer's disease, a vascular dementia, or a less common entity, some aspects of mental status must be impaired for dementia to be present. Loss of memory for recent events, impaired judgment, inability to concentrate, and loss of abstract reasoning are some of the mental status deficits commonly seen.

No measure of mental status is perfect. In research, the best available method for determining mental status is a detailed psychiatric interview. As is more commonly done, our study employed a standardized questionnaire to estimate the degree of mental status impairment.

Measurement of Mental Status

Eight questions that comprise the mental status portion of the MOSES were used to measure mental status. The eight items are: understanding communication, talking, way finding, recognizing staff, awareness of place, awareness of time, recent memory, and past memory. When residents do not verbalize, items that require verbalization, such as awareness of time, are omitted. All items are rated on a four-point scale, with 1 representing no impairment and 4, severe impairment. A summary scale

TABLE 4.6   Communication Skills of Residents

	Dementia Unit Residents[a]	Comparison Unit Residents[a]	Chi-square[b]	p
Understanding communication (speaking, writing, or gesturing)				
Understood clearly	28.3%	30.2%	2.4	.49
Understood only brief communications	28.0	26.4		
Understood only if repeated	30.6	26.7		
Did not understand	13.2	16.7		
Spoken communication				
Coherent and logical	15.3	22.0	9.2	.06
Wandered off topic	26.1	19.2		
Sounded coherent but was irrelevant	22.5	18.2		
Made very little sense	26.1	29.2		
Did not speak	10.1	11.3		

[a]Dementia unit sample size was 304 subjects for understanding communication and 307 for spoken communication. Comparison unit sample size was 318 for both items.
[b]Three degrees of freedom for understanding communication; four degrees of freedom for spoken communication.

is then constructed by computing the mean of all the items for which a score was available and multiplying the result by 100. That summary score ranges from 100 to 400.

This measure of mental status is indirect. It depends on rating by a staff member who knows the resident well. Direct measures of mental status, such as the Short Portable Mental Status Questionnaire (Pfeiffer 1975) and the Folstein Mini-Mental State Examination (Folstein et al. 1975), were not used. As is noted in the Appendix, our study did not use measures that involve speaking with or examining the subjects. This avoided the need to obtain individual informed consent, but it limited our ability to measure cognitive status.

Mental Status Measures in Dementia Units and Comparison Units

Difficulty remembering recent events is the single most widely recognized sign of mental status impairment. In our dementia unit sample, 97 percent of subjects were identified as having some impairment of

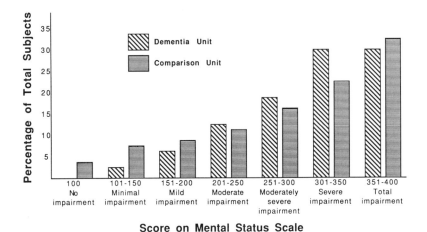

FIGURE 4.3   Mental status of residents: dementia units versus comparison units.

recent memory, as opposed to 87.5 percent of comparison unit subjects. This difference is statistically significant ($p < .001$). Comparative data from the 1985 National Nursing Home Survey showed 75.8 percent of people identified as having "senile dementia/chronic and organic brain syndrome" had disorientation or memory impairment to the degree that they were "impaired nearly every day in performing the basic activities of daily living, mobility, and adaptive tasks." Of those without such a diagnosis, 25.9 percent had disorientation or memory impairment.

Using the scale computed from MOSES mental status items, the overall mean mental status score was 303. The mean for dementia units was 310; the mean for comparison units was 296. This difference, while small, was statistically significant ($p = .031$). Thus, dementia units on average appear to manage residents whose mental status is slightly more impaired than comparison units.

When the actual scores are compared on a frequency bar chart (figure 4.3), it is apparent that this difference in mean mental status scores arises because the comparison units had more residents with little or no mental status impairment. Two explanations for this observation exist: either (1) comparison units serve a wider range of dementia residents, including those in very early phases of the disease who may have been institutionalized for other reasons than their dementing illness; or (2) some people in comparison units labeled as having a dementia diagnosis may not have a progressive mental disorder such as Alzheimer's disease and, in fact, may not have a chronic dementing disorder at all.

The Relationship between Mental Status and Communication Skills

When we compared the scores on communication skills with mental status scores, we discovered that the two measures were colinear. While some association was expected because the two communication items are a subset of the eight-item mental status score, the magnitude of the association was surprising. When the mental status index (scaled from 100 to 400) was plotted against the communication index (scaled from 200 to 900), a near-perfect linear association was observed. The Pearson correlation coefficient between the two variables was .820, again confirming the strong link between mental status and communication.

This finding suggests a direct relationship between deterioration in mental status and loss of communication skills. It also suggests that whatever process leads to impairment of memory and other mental status parameters may affect communication in a similar manner and by a similar mechanism. Since communication is an important and readily measurable characteristic, it may represent the mental status measure that is most meaningful in the nursing home.

Behavioral Problems

While mental status impairment is the ubiquitous feature of Alzheimer's disease and related disorders, behavioral problems are the most troublesome issue for the staff. Screaming, wandering, agitation, disturbing other's belongings, noncooperation with caregivers, socially inappropriate behavior such as disrobing in public, verbal outbursts, and physical abusiveness are among the problem behaviors staff must manage. Behavior problems are not limited to people with dementia, but they occur far more commonly in this group. According to our analyses of 1985 National Nursing Home Survey data, for example, physically abusive behavior is 2.3 times more common among residents who have a dementia diagnosis than those not afflicted with these disorders. Our study used the MOSES, the Resource Utilization Groups (RUGs) resident classification system, and our structured observations of residents to gather data on behavioral problems.

IDENTIFICATION OF PROBLEM BEHAVIORS

The MOSES questionnaire, which was completed on each resident by a staff member contained an eight-item behavioral problem inventory. Items 25 through 32 on the MOSES rated the following behaviors: cooperation with nursing care, following staff requests and instructions, irritability, reactions to frustration, verbal abuse of staff, verbal abuse of other residents, physical abuse of others, and provoking arguments with other residents. Each item was rated on a four-point scale, with 1 indicating no problem and 4 indicating a frequent problem. Some of the items had an additional "not ratable" score for instances when the resident could not manifest the behavior (such as verbal abusiveness) because of aphasia.

The MOSES subscale for behavioral problems is constructed by computing the mean score for these eight items, omitting the questions that were not ratable. Using this system and multiplying the result by 100 yielded a continuous variable ranging between 100 and 400. From this, we divided the residents into three categories: no problems (scores less than 200); minor problems (scores between 200 and 299); and major problems (scores of 300 or greater). We also performed analyses based on only two categories: without major behavioral problems (scores of 250 or lower); and with major behavioral problems (scores above 250).

The RUGs scores, which were computed separately on the basis of staff interview or (in New York) taken directly from the medical record, contain a separate category for residents exhibiting major behavioral problems. To be placed in that category, a resident had to exhibit a major disruptive behavior such as physical abusiveness, smearing feces on walls, or severe agitation at least once a week for the prior month.

Finally, during our structured observations of individual residents, overt behavioral problems were noted. These included moaning, crying or screaming, talking to self, physically aggressive or quarrelsome behavior, tenseness, wandering, pounding tables or trays, and other signs of agitation or aggressiveness.

COMPARATIVE FREQUENCIES OF BEHAVIORAL PROBLEMS IN DEMENTIA UNITS AND COMPARISON UNITS

Overall, the proportion of residents exhibiting behavioral problems was similar in the two settings but slightly higher on the dementia units. Analysis of individual behavioral items on the MOSES revealed no significant difference between dementia units and comparison units in cooperation with nursing care, following staff requests, irritability, or verbal abusiveness toward staff. Dementia units reported slightly more problems with provoking arguments, exhibiting frustration reactions, verbal abusiveness toward other residents, and physical abusiveness. For each of these behaviors, the major difference was a higher frequency of occasional problems; frequent problems occurred no more often in dementia units than in comparison units.

When the MOSES questions were aggregated into a summary behavioral scale, dementia unit scores were slightly higher, but the difference was not statistically significant. The mean score for the 307 dementia unit residents was 184; the mean for the 317 comparison unit residents rated was 177 ($p = .21$, not significant).

A separate section of the MOSES asked whether the resident showed signs of anxiety, worry, or fear. The findings did not indicate significant differences between settings. In dementia units, 18 percent of residents exhibited signs of anxiety or worry; in comparison units, the proportion was 15 percent ($p = .29$, not significant).

This trend for dementia units to demonstrate a slight but statistically insignificant increase in behavioral problems also occurred in the RUGs scores. Twenty-four percent of dementia unit residents were classified in the RUGs behavioral problems category, compared with 19 percent of comparison unit residents. That difference was not statistically significant ($p = .10$, not significant).

When we made individual observations on residents during our nonparticipant observation, we also observed a slight but statistically insignificant increase in behavioral problems among dementia unit residents. Overall, 24 percent of dementia unit residents exhibited one or more problem behaviors during our brief observation, compared with 19 percent of comparison unit residents ($p = .12$, not significant). We noted slightly more moaning and screaming (4.7 versus 2.6 percent of subjects) on comparison units, and more wandering (6.9 versus 3.8 percent of subjects) on dementia units, but neither difference was statistically significant.

Interpretation of these observations is difficult. It is apparent that dementia units do not manage fewer residents with behavioral problems than do comparison units; in fact they appear to manage a higher proportion of such residents. The relatively high proportion of mild problems reported by the dementia units may reflect a staff that is more attuned to such issues and, therefore, reports them more frequently. On the other hand, since all measures showed a trend for problem behaviors to be higher in dementia units, we believe that this difference, though small, is valid.

What we are unable to estimate is the effect of the setting itself on behaviors. If dementia units admit a higher proportion of individuals with problem behaviors, as some units claim, they may be managing those behaviors much better than the comparison units. If the entry characteristics of both groups of residents are similar, then control of problem behaviors is no better on dementia units. Only a longitudinal prospective study, preferably with randomization, could separate the effects of entry characteristics and treatment.

LIMITATIONS OF OUR BEHAVIORAL PROBLEM MEASURES

As we visited nursing homes, spoke with staff, and observed the residents in our study, we began to feel that established measures of behavioral problems may not be sensitive enough to detect differences in nursing care requirements. All our measures looked for overt problems, such as physical abusiveness in the past week or agitation on direct observation. If a behavior was controlled, but it took extra staff effort to control it, our measures categorized the resident as having no behavioral problems.

This issue came to our attention while we visited nursing homes in New York State, whose case-mix reimbursement uses the RUGs to determine payment rates. As discussed above, the RUGs places residents with overt behavioral problems in a separate category. Reimbursement for these residents is higher than for similar residents without behavioral problems. On several occasions, administrators of dementia units commented that the reimbursement system punished them for controlling problem behaviors. The resident who could be behaviorally controlled with extra staff effort was not identified as a behavioral problem and reimbursement was the same as for a nondemented resident with similar ADL status.

In fact, while it is not considered an overt behavioral issue, proper care of dementia residents often requires more time for grooming, bathing, and virtually every staff task. Many of these people must be approached cautiously, must have procedures carefully explained, and require extra supervision to achieve maximum independence. The impact of these more subtle behavioral issues on nursing staff time is an area needing further study.

Nursing Care Requirements: The RUGs Scores

The Resource Utilization Groups (RUGs) resident classification system places each resident in 1 of 16 categories. The data used to assign resident scores are: the intensiveness of nursing procedures required, the presence or absence of severe behavioral problems, and scores on three activities of daily living (feeding, transfer, and continence). Each RUGs category contains residents whose nursing care requirements are relatively homogeneous. A number of states use the RUGs system to determine reimbursement.

We calculated RUGs scores for all subjects in the study except those in New York, where the scores were available on resident medical records. The results are contained in table 4.7, along with comparison data for all nursing home residents in New York and Texas. Both of our study samples have similar RUGs profiles, with few residents receiving highly technical nursing care or rehabilitation (RUGs scores 1 to 8) and a relatively high proportion of residents in the behavioral problem categories (RUGs scores 9 to 11), when compared with all nursing home residents. There was a tendency for comparison unit residents to be concentrated in

TABLE 4.7 Resource Utilization Groups (RUG-II) Categorization of Study Subjects, with Comparison Estimates for All Nursing Home Residents in New York and Texas (%)

RUG-II Category	In Dementia Units	In Comparison Units	All Nursing Home Residents[a] New York	Texas
1. Special A	0	0	1.5	1.0
2. Special B	1.3	2.8	5.7	5.8
3. Rehabilitation A	0	0	2.0	0
4. Rehabilitation B	0	1.3	3.6	0.9
5. Clinically complex A	0.7	0.3	3.9	4.7
6. Clinically complex B	0.3	1.3	6.6	8.6
7. Clinically complex C	1.6	2.2	4.8	8.7
8. Clinically complex D	0	2.5	1.0	1.0
9. Severe behavorial A	3.0	2.8	3.2	2.4
10. Severe behavioral B	17.2	9.7	7.9	5.9
11. Severe behavioral C	4.0	6.3	3.7	2.2
12. Physical A	18.2	12.0	25.9	25.2
13. Physical B	10.9	2.5	3.0	2.4
14. Physical C	26.1	30.9	19.5	21.9
15. Physical D	7.3	10.4	6.2	7.4
16. Physical E	9.6	15.1	1.4	2.0

[a]Unpublished data courtesy of Brant Fries, Ph.D., University of Michigan.

the more physically impaired categories, particularly in RUGs scores 15 and 16. On the other hand, as we discussed earlier in this chapter, dementia units contained a larger proportion of people with scores indicating severe behavioral problems, but that difference did not achieve statistical significance.

Family Visitation

Families can provide important emotional support for nursing home residents. By entertaining on their own or participating in activities, family members can provide extra attention and stimulation for a loved one. How often family members visit depends on both the strength of family bonds, the ability of family members to visit, and the degree to which a facility makes family members feel welcome.

Our pilot studies had shown that family visits were frequently not

TABLE 4.8 Frequency of Visits by Any Family Member (%)

Frequency	Dementia Unit Residents (N = 314)	Comparison Unit Residents (N = 307)
Two or more times a week	41.7	33.5
About once a week	18.9	21.5
Less than once a week but more than once a month	17.9	13.6
Once a month or less	21.5	31.3

Note: $p = .01$. The frequency of visits was estimated by the nursing staff.

recorded by nursing staff. Therefore, we measured family visitation rates for each study subject by asking nursing staff how often family members had visited the resident during the past month. We asked several staff members at the same time. In that way they could share the information they had, and we could obtain the most accurate information possible.

We found that residents on dementia units had higher family visitation rates than those on our comparison units. In dementia units, 41.7 percent of residents had two or more family visits a week, compared with 33.5 percent of residents of comparison units. In contrast, comparison units had a higher proportion of family members who seldom or never visited (31.3 versus 21.5 percent). Table 4.8 displays these findings; its results are statistically significant ($p = .01$).

Comparison of Dementia Units in Proprietary and Nonprofit Homes

When we planned this study, we were encouraged to examine whether dementia units in proprietary (for-profit) homes serve a different population than those in nonprofit homes. A number of for-profit nursing home chains have made concerted efforts to build dementia units. They have been criticized as being highly selective of the type of resident they accept, seeking out people in the early stages of dementia with private pay resources and with relatively low nursing care needs. To test this hypothesis, we analyzed several variables to look for differences between the proprietary and nonprofit dementia units we visited. Table 4.9 summarizes the results of these analyses.

Overall, we noted very little difference between the residents in proprietary and those in nonprofit dementia units. The for-profit units have a slightly younger population with a shorter mean length of stay, perhaps reflecting in part the fact that the proprietary units we visited were newer on average than the nonprofit units. Gender, marital status, race, comorbidity, payment status, mental status, ADL dependency, and behavioral problem scores did not differ between the two groups. Thus, little or no difference exists between the residents of for-profit and non-profit dementia units.

Degree of Variation in Dementia Populations of Individual Homes

Because we visited a wide variety of units in many different homes and studied 10 residents at each site, observed differences among the resident populations could be due to random chance alone. In contrast, we were aware that certain units by policy or certification either exclude or solicit residents with certain characteristics. We were also aware that each facility had its own "atmosphere" or "feeling," some of which was created by its mix of residents. In an attempt to capture and describe this variation among dementia populations in various nursing home units, we studied interunit variability for selected resident characteristics.

The variables we studied were three eight-item indexes from the MOSES: the ADL Score, the mental status index, and the behavioral problems index. For each variable, we plotted individual and mean scores, looking for differences between states, between proprietary and non-proprietary homes, and between units certified at skilled and those at intermediate levels, as well as for facilities that were outliers. The significant differences we observed are summarized below.

ACTIVITIES OF DAILY LIVING

Mean ADL scores for individual units varied between 205 and 380. No outliers were noted. There was no overall difference in ADL status between dementia units and comparison units. Within California and Ohio, however, dementia unit residents tended to have fewer ADL impairments than residents in matched comparison units. Among the dementia units visited, those in New York tended to have residents with the greatest ADL impairment, those in Texas the least. As expected, the greatest differences in ADL status were observed when skilled facilities were compared with intermediate facilities; ADL impairments were significantly higher in skilled facilities.

MENTAL STATUS

Mean scores on mental status for individual units ranged between 235 and 355. One comparison unit in Texas was an outlier, with a mean

TABLE 4.9   Comparison of Proprietary and Nonprofit Dementia Units

	Proprietary (150 residents in 15 units)	Nonprofit (147 residents in 15 units)	p^*
Mean age of dementia unit (yr)	3.1	6.0	n.s.
Mean resident age (yr)	78.8	81.4	<.01
Mean no. of days since this admission (LOS-A)	538	653	n.s.
Mean no. of days in any nursing home (LOS-NH)	784	890	n.s.
Married with living spouse (%)	21	26	n.s.
Female (%)	77	73	n.s.
Private payment status (%)	59	61	n.s.
Race/ethnicity (%)			
White	94	97	n.s.
Black	5	3	
Hispanic	1	1	
History (%)			
Stroke	5	5	n.s.
Hip fracture	7	13	n.s.
Other fracture	2	1	n.s.
Current condition (%)			
Cardiovascular medication	49	37	<.05
Visual impairment	14	12	n.s.
Hearing impairment (deafness)	1	4	.05
Mean communication score	517	509	n.s.
Mean ADL score	276	289	n.s.
Mean summary behavorial problem score	178	192	n.s.

*Chi-square used to test for differences in percentages, t test for differences in means; n.s., not significant.

score of 210, indicating less impaired residents. No significant associations were noted between mental status and state, ownership, level of care, or whether the unit was specialized or not. When the communication skills variable was examined independently, residents of intermediate care facilities were seen to have better scores.

BEHAVIORAL PROBLEMS

Mean scores for behavioral problems ranged between 130 and 245. One comparison unit in New York was an outlier, with a score of 275.

TABLE 4.10 A Comparison of Residents Aged 65 and Older in Four Settings (%)

Site[a]	Mean Age (yr)	Older than Age 84	Female	White	Married	Dependent in Dressing	Bathing	Transfer	Incontinent
Community[b]	73.4	7.2	59.2	90.5	55.1	4.3	5.9	2.8	9.0
Adult day care[c]	77.7	19.6	63.8	73.3	28.9	35.4	45.8	23.2	14.9
Specialized dementia units	81.1	40.6	75.5	94.8	23.4	81.4	93.1	46.6	69.1
All nursing home residents[d]	83.0	45.3	74.7	93.1	13.0	77.4	90.3	61.8	51.7

[a]For standardization, only people past age 64 are included.
[b]Source: 1984 National Health Interview Survey's Supplement on Aging.
[c]Source: survey data collected by Weissert et al. (1989).
[d]Source: 1985 National Nursing Home Survey.

Otherwise, no significant trends were noted between behavioral problems and state, ownership, or level of care.

Summary: Who Resides in Dementia Units?

Specialized dementia units serve people who are predominantly elderly and demented, with Alzheimer's disease the most prevalent diagnosis. Overall, these units contain a population that is younger, more mobile, and less incontinent; requires less care with dressing; and has a slightly higher prevalence of behavioral problems than demented residents of integrated units. They discharge residents home or to other nursing home units more frequently than integrated units and provide terminal care only infrequently.

Table 4.10 compares our findings on residents in dementia units with similar data for community elderly, adult day care residents, and all nursing home residents. These results suggest that dementia unit residents occupy a position intermediate in many respects between people in adult day care and the average nursing home resident. Age, marital status, and mobility impairment, as represented by ability to transfer, clearly show similar trends. Several factors could contribute to such a finding, including the documented newness of many units, differences in selecting residences for dementia units when compared with traditional units, improved quality of care on dementia units, and selective discharge policies on the part of the dementia units.

Certain impairments particularly characteristic of dementing illness are, however, more common among dementia unit residents than nursing home residents in general (see table 4.10). These include dependency in dressing, continence, and bathing. Thus, dementia units do appear to serve a unique population with certain dependencies and problems characteristic of dementing illnesses.

References

Folstein, M. F., Folstein, S., and McHugh, P. H. 1975. Mini-mental state: Practical method for grading cognitive state of patients for the clinician. *Journal of Psychiatric Research* 12: 189–98.

Helmes, E., Csapo, K. G., and Short, J. A. 1987. Standardization and Validation of the Multidimensional Observation Scale for Elderly Subjects (MOSES). *Journal of Gerontology* 42: 395–405.

Pfeiffer, E. 1975. A short portable mental status questionnaire for the assessment of organic brain deficit in elderly patients. *Journal of the American Geriatrics Society* 23: 433–41.

Weissert, W. G., et al. 1989. Models of adult day care: Findings from a national survey. *Gerontologist* 29: 640–49.

5

Assessing the Resident with Dementia

PHILIP D. SLOANE AND LAURA J. MATHEW

Nursing home residents with dementia vary widely in needs and abilities. For staff who provide care for such persons, accurate and meaningful assessment is crucial to planning appropriate services. Individualization is important, but of equal value is the ability to place dementia residents in meaningful categories for admission, program planning, and evaluation purposes. This chapter briefly highlights some of the literature on classification of people with dementia. Then it proposes an approach to assessment that helps identify care priorities for dementia residents in nursing homes.

Common Diagnoses among Residents of Dementia Units

Much of the literature on assessment and classification of people with dementia deals solely with Alzheimer's disease. Only about two-thirds of dementia residents in nursing homes have pure Alzheimer's disease. Most of the remainder have either multi-infarct dementia or both Alzheimer's and multi-infarct disease. A few have Parkinson's disease, dementia secondary to chronic alcoholism, normal pressure hydrocephalus, Huntington's disease, or some other less common cause of brain impairment. Among nursing home residents, nonspecific diagnoses, such as "organic brain syndrome" or "chronic confusion," are common.

Clinically, typical Alzheimer's disease and multi-infarct dementia are somewhat different. Alzheimer's disease is thought to represent a slow but continuous deterioration of brain cells. Multi-infarct disease, on the other hand, results from a series of small strokes in the brain, with no additional deterioration occurring between strokes. Thus, Alzheimer's disease is said to progress gradually, whereas multi-infarct dementia progresses in a stepwise fashion. In addition, people with multi-infarct disease more often have gait problems early in the disease and are said to be more emotionally labile (emotional incontinence).

In practice, however, it is difficult to make a precise diagnosis. What usually happens in academic centers is that a series of laboratory tests are done, including either computerized scanning (CAT) or magnetic imaging (MRI) of the brain. If signs of previous stroke are evident, then multi-infarct disease is diagnosed. If tests indicate a rarer disease, such as parkinsonism, central nervous system syphilis, or normal pressure hydrocephalus, that disease is diagnosed. If all tests are negative, then a presumptive diagnosis of Alzheimer's disease is made. Autopsy studies show, however, that our current methods of diagnosis are not always accurate.

From a caregiving perspective, the actual diagnosis makes little difference, so long as treatable disorders and secondary causes of disability have been ruled out or treated. Staff should assess all dementia residents directly rather than draw inferences from the diagnosis. A single approach can be used to evaluate all demented residents.

STAGING IN ALZHEIMER'S DISEASE

Several systems have been proposed to stage Alzheimer's disease. Gwyther and Matteson (1983) described a three-stage model; Glickstein (1988) identified four stages. The most detailed work has been done by Reisberg (1983, 1984), who identified seven stages of cognitive decline in elderly patients. His seven levels, briefly, are:

1. Normal—no cognitive changes.
2. Normal aged forgetfulness—difficulty remembering names and where things were placed, but no interferences with social, work, or home activities.
3. Early confusion—memory loss that begins to interfere with life activities, often accompanied by anxiety.
4. Late confusion—loss of ability to handle routine matters such as shopping and finances, and minimal disorientation, accompanied frequently by a denial defense response, and emotional withdrawal.

5. Early dementia—frequent disorientation; difficulty with simple tasks such as choosing clothes or bathing; differing levels of function from day to day and within one day; anger, suspicion, and transient crying episodes.

6. Middle dementia—fragmentary memory; fear of bathing; decline in memory of simple processes requiring step-by-step instructions and assistance in later stages for activities such as toileting; incontinence (frequently); fear of the world, commonly accompanied by agitation and paranoia.

7. Late dementia—gradual loss of ability to perform basic body functions, such as walking and feeding; decline in verbal skill until few or no words are spoken, although the ability to smile or laugh may remain; a passive mood in spite of anger and resistance to care.

Because institutionalization usually occurs during stage 5, most Alzheimer's residents in nursing homes are in the last three stages.

Other studies have documented the fact that Alzheimer's disease and related illnesses follow an unpredictable pattern. For example, one person may retain excellent verbal and social abilities, while another at the same functional level may speak only a few repetitive words. Some of these differences in patterns of dysfunction can be explained by focal strokes (coexisting multi-infarct disease), but even pure Alzheimer's patients vary widely. Jorm (1985) reported that Alzheimer's disease is sometimes but not always characterized by early language disturbance, which is at times an indicator of familial disease. Suspiciousness and restlessness are not related to the stage of the disease, but decline in personal hygiene, agitation, and wandering become more common as mental status deteriorates (Teri et al. 1988). According to Jackson et al. (1989), the most prevalent disruptive behaviors in nursing homes are abusiveness, noisiness, and wandering. Wandering is most common in the ambulatory confused, noisiness among the late-stage demented, and abusive behaviors at all ADL levels.

RESIDENT ASSESSMENT

Evaluation of a resident with dementia by nursing home staff should address those behaviors that are most vital to daily life in the home. It should also identify individual strengths and weaknesses. Ultimately, a proper assessment helps staff set priorities and goals.

Dementia residents should be evaluated for activities of daily living, behavioral problems, communication abilities, and physical transition status (Sloane and Mathew 1990). These four categories, which are crucial because they allow nursing home staff to determine general care priorities and approaches, are discussed below. Table 5.1 presents the profile

TABLE 5.1   Proportion of Residents in Each Assessment Category (%)

Category	In Dementia Units (N = 307)	In Comparison Units (N = 318)
ADL status		
Ambulatory confused	46.9	21.2
Failing in transfer, ambulation, continence, or feeding	39.6	55.4
Late stage	13.5	23.4
Special behavioral problems		
Major behavioral problems present (e.g., abusiveness, severe agitation, infantile or socially inappropriate behavior	34.0	30.1
No major disruptive behaviors	36.0	69.9
Communication impairment		
None or minor	27.0	29.2
Moderate	26.1	23.9
Severe	46.9	46.9
In physical transition		
Recent admission (< 1 month ago)	4.9	2.2
Unstable medical problems	2.6	5.7
Both recent admission and instability	1.4	0.6
Not in physical transition	91.1	91.5

of our dementia unit and comparison unit study subjects in these four areas.

Activities of Daily Living

Activities of Daily Living (ADLs) are basic life tasks, such as bathing, dressing, grooming, transferring from bed to chair, walking or wheeling independently, and feeding. Among residents in the later stages of dementia, special attention should be given to feeding and mobility (range of motion of arms and legs, ability to transfer and ambulate, and ability to shift position in a chair or in bed). Each of these activities should be evaluated in terms of what the resident can do and how much assistance is required for adequate performance. Dementia residents can be divided into three ADL subgroups based on their ability to transfer, ambulate, and remain continent.

Residents in the most independent ADL category can ambulate, transfer from a bed to a chair, eat, and use the bathroom either by themselves or with reminders. They represented 46.9 percent of dementia unit residents and about 21.2 percent of comparison unit residents (table 5.1). For these *ambulatory confused*, the top priority in care planning is independence and involvement, with an intense, appropriate therapeutic activity program comprising the most beneficial care modality.

The middle group in ADL function have some impairment of transfer, ambulation, or continence but are not yet totally dependent in these areas. They constituted 39.6 percent of dementia unit residents and 55.4 percent of comparison unit residents. Such people, who are said to be *failing*, require a particularly well coordinated effort between activities and nursing, with maintenance of mobility the primary treatment goal.

At the most impaired end of the spectrum are the *late-stage* residents, who have lost control over virtually all body functions. These composed 13.5 percent of dementia unit residents and 23.4 percent of comparison unit residents. Help is needed with feeding (initially, some can still feed themselves); urinary (and often fecal) incontinence is present; and the resident is largely confined to a bed or a chair. At this stage of illness, nursing care needs take priority over activities or programming. Because these residents require several hours of direct nursing attention daily, high-quality nursing is the most important component of their care. Nevertheless, they often respond to a variety of treatments, including direct physical contact with caregivers, certain favorite foods, and music. Goals for late-stage residents revolve around comfort, contact, preservation of dignity, and maintenance of basic body integrity.

Behavioral Problems

Certain behavioral disruptions require a specific plan on the part of the nursing home staff; if not controlled, they interfere with functioning of the unit. Such problems, while not uncommon, go beyond the disorientation and resistance to certain care activities (like bathing) seen in nearly all dementia residents. Wandering into other's rooms, repeated verbal challenges to others, verbal or physical abusiveness, public disrobing or sexual behavior, and severe agitation outbursts are typical examples. Among our study subjects, 34.0 percent of dementia unit residents and 30.1 percent of comparison unit residents were identified as having major behavioral problems by either the RUGs or the MOSES (see chapter 4).

People with severe disruptive behavior make it difficult to pursue the goals of care and often disrupt the entire unit. For such people, a primary goal of treatment has to be effective control of the problem behavior. Behavioral control facilitates the achievement of other care goals, such as support of ADLs and involvement in activities.

Communication Skills

The ability to understand verbal or written information, the ability to speak or write, and use of nonverbal communication are communication skills. More impaired people communicate through facial expressions; moans, screams, and other utterances; or body movements. Among our study subjects, 27.0 percent of dementia unit residents and 29.2 percent of comparison unit residents had mild communication problems, as defined by a score of 399 or lower on the index of communication skills (see fig. 4.2); 26.1 percent of dementia unit residents and 23.9 percent of comparison unit residents had moderate problems (index scores of 400 to 599); and 46.9 percent of both dementia unit residents and comparison unit residents had severe impairment (scores of 600 and above).

People who communicate well verbally do better in group activities; those with more limited communication skills need more one-to-one attention. Use of written signs is another ability that depends on communication skills; some people can read and repeat but do not comprehend words such as "rest room"; others can use such cues. Part of the assessment of communication involves identifying hearing or visual problems, which on their own can impair communication.

Physical Transition

Newly arrived residents (those in the first month after admission) and those who are currently being treated for an acute illness tend to have rapidly changing needs and abilities. Recent admissions are at unusually high risk for falls and injury, changes in medical and behavioral status, hospitalization, and death. New admissions also include residents most likely to return home or to be rehabilitated to a less intensive level of care. Similarly, people being treated for acute medical problems, such as pneumonia, tend to experience rapid change. These residents are at particular risk of new functional problems, such as skin breakdown, fecal impaction, contractures, or oversedation, particularly if nursing staff fail to recognize and adjust their care to accommodate the resident's increased dependency. For these reasons, people in physical transition should receive special attention directed toward detecting new problems and changing care needs. Assessment must be frequent, and changing needs reflected in altered care plans.

Setting Care Priorities

On the basis of these four areas (a convenient mnemonic is ABC-T), nursing home staff can rapidly identify priorities in caring for residents with Alzheimer's disease and related disorders. Staff can also identify to what extent nursing care and activities should take the lead in case man-

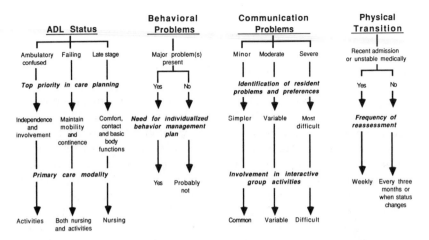

FIGURE 5.1   Essential assessment areas and their implications for planning care. ADL, activities of daily living.

agement; the likelihood that a person will do well in groups; the frequency of reassessment that is likely to be needed; and overall goals for care. Figure 5.1 summarizes this process.

ADDITIONAL ASSESSMENT AREAS

Three additional areas are important to evaluate if assessment is to be reasonably complete. These are medical status, mood, and social and activity preferences.

Medical Status

A medical evaluation is necessary to confirm that dementia is present, to rule out treatable causes of the dementia, and to look for other medical problems that may complicate the resident's status. For example, while nursing home residents with dementia are rarely cured, a number of treatable diseases can mimic dementia. These include delirium (a state of confusion that can be caused by drugs, metabolic problems, or any acute illness) and depression. Furthermore, care planning must also consider the existence of treatable illnesses or disabilities, such as chronic lung disease or a recent hip fracture. Discussing the resident's status with knowledgeable family members and the attending physician, combined with a review of the medical record, gives the most complete portrait of the resident's medical status.

Mood

Anxiety, depression, agitation, withdrawal, and lability are among the mood disturbances frequently seen in dementing illness. Withdrawn and passive residents are especially susceptible to being neglected, thereby declining more rapidly than necessary in social skills, strength, mobility, and often nutrition. Occasionally, a problem such as severe depression improves with medication. More commonly, staff must adjust their approach to accommodate the resident's mood.

Social and Activity Preferences

A variety of factors should be considered here, including: preference of a single room versus one with a roommate, degree of interest and participation in group activities, interest in the opposite sex versus same sex, racial or other preferences (and prejudices), responsiveness to one-to-one verbal activities, response to touch and other physical communication by staff and other residents, type of personal space desired and response to infringements, and types of activities preferred. Chapters 12 and 13 discuss in detail the assessment of individual activity preferences.

FROM ASSESSMENT TO CAREGIVING

The precise method by which a nursing home assesses its residents is up to the individual institution. A variety of instruments have been developed, such as the MOSES (Helmes et al. 1987), to evaluate these areas. Many nursing homes and corporations have developed their own assessment systems. Recently, as a provision of the Nursing Home Reform Act of 1987, the Health Care Financing Administration has developed a standardized assessment instrument, the Minimum Data Set (Morris et al. 1990), which assesses the above areas and may prove helpful to nursing home staff.

More important than the actual assessment method is the use of assessment data to develop care plans that identify priorities in ways that help staff. There is always more that can be done for residents than staff can accomplish. Without a sense of priorities, staff members feel overloaded and can become frustrated. Finally, without a consensus on what the goals and priorities are, staff members do not work together. For example, a new admission who is able to walk but is weak and incontinent will be easier to toilet if her ambulatory status can be improved. Staff should understand that walking her should be a top priority, and that achieving continence will be emphasized once she can walk better.

Resident care conferences in which all disciplines participate provide the best method of reviewing assessment information and developing realistic care plans. If they have had an opportunity to share in the planning, all staff better appreciate and are better prepared to provide high-quality care.

References

Glickstein, J. K. 1988. *Therapeutic Interventions in Alzheimer's Disease: A Program of Functional Communication Skills for Activities of Daily Living.* Rockville, Md: Aspen.

Gwyther, L., and Matteson, M. A. 1983. Care for the caregivers. *Journal of Gerontological Nursing* 9: 92–95, 100, 116.

Helmes, E., Csapo, K. G., and Short, J. A. 1987. Standardization and validation of the Multidimensional Observation Scale for Elderly Subjects (moses). *Journal of Gerontology* 42: 395–405.

Jackson, M. E., et al. 1989. Prevalence and correlates of disruptive behavior in the nursing home. *Journal of Aging and Health* 1: 349–69.

Jorm, A. F. 1985. Subtypes of Alzheimer's dementia: A conceptual analysis and critical review. *Psychological Medicine* 15: 543–53.

Morris, J. M., et al. 1990. Designing the national resident assessment instrument for nursing homes. *Gerontologist* 30: 293–307.

Reisberg, B. 1983. Clinical presentation, diagnosis, and symptomatology of age-associated cognitive decline and Alzheimer's disease. In R. Reisberg (ed.), *Alzheimer's Disease.* New York: Free Press.

———1984. Stages of cognitive decline. *American Journal of Nursing* 84: 225–28.

Sloane, P. D., and Mathew, L. J. 1991. An assessment and care-planning strategy for nursing home residents with dementia. *Gerontologist,* 31: 128–31.

Teri, L., Larson, E. B., and Reifler, B. V. 1988. Behavioral disturbance in dementia of the Alzheimer's type. *Journal of the American Geriatrics Society* 36: 1–6.

III

Organization and Staffing

6

Organizing and Staffing Dementia Units

LAURA J. MATHEW AND PHILIP D. SLOANE

Although some universal characteristics of dementia units have been described in the literature (Weiner and Reingold 1989), administrators continue to use a variety of approaches. Reasons for this include a lack of uniform standards, debate over the types of residents most likely to benefit from special programming, and a lack of agreement about what program elements are most therapeutic. The type of staff and the staff–resident ratios needed to care for this unique population have also not been adequately researched. As a result, facilities use a number of strategies and very often reflect their own institutional policies in these matters. New units of large nursing home chains usually follow a set of guidelines that have been predetermined by consultants of the corporation. These variations in program design are healthy and expected, since much is still to be determined about optimal care for residents with dementia.

This chapter describes administrative issues and the manner in which the 31 specialized dementia units we visited handled them. It presents and discusses data regarding admission and discharge policies, unit size, and certification level. In addition, services provided to the community, involvement with dementia research, and service as a site for student learning are discussed. Finally, staffing issues are described: staffing ratios, turnover rates, and services provided for the staff. Where appropriate, parallels are made between the dementia units and comparison units. For details of the study design, please see the introduction and Appendix.

Admissions and Discharges to the Units

Our administrative questionnaire contained seven questions relating to admission and discharge routines. Items included whether or not the unit had a waiting list, the average waiting time in months, how potential dementia unit participants were screened, the percentage of in-house transfers, whether or not residents were divided into groups, how often residents were discharged to a lower (or less intensive) level of care, and the actual number of residents discharged to a lower level of care.

Most dementia units (63.3 percent) stated that they had a waiting list; about one-third (36.7 percent) did not. The average time patients had to wait for admission to a unit was 3.8 months. The range was wide; some units reported no time spent awaiting a bed, and one unit had an average wait of 17 months.

Residents were screened in several ways (see table 6.1). No dementia unit used only a questionnaire to screen potential participants. The largest percentage (50 percent) stated that they used both a questionnaire and a personal visit. An additional 13.3 percent stated that they used not only a questionnaire and a personal visit, but some other method of screening. A few (6.7 percent) used a personal visit by itself. About 20 percent used a personal visit and some other method, and only 10 percent used only some other method of screening participants.

All dementia units were asked about the likelihood that residents from within their own facility would be transferred to the unit. The estimated percentage of in-house transfers ranged from 0 to 100. Units who admitted 27 percent or fewer of their residents from within their own facility were regrouped into a category defined as having most admissions coming from outside. Those with more than 27 percent of admissions as in-house transfers were defined as looking within the facility for admissions. Forty percent of the units we sampled accepted largely in-house transfers. Sixty percent admitted a substantial proportion of their residents from outside the facility.

The tendency to attract outside admissions did not seem to vary by ownership status or size of the home. About 46.7 percent of the nonprofit homes fell into the category of admitting most of their participants from within the facility, and about 33.3 percent of the for-profit homes fit this description. Table 6.2 lists these figures; the differences were not statis-

TABLE 6.1   Methods Used to Screen Admissions (%)

Method	Dementia Units (N = 30)
Questionnaire alone	0
Personal visit alone	6.7
Questionnaire and personal visit	50.0
Questionnaire, personal visit, and another method	13.3
Personal visit and another method	20.0
Another method	10.0

TABLE 6.2   Origin of Admissions to Nonprofit and For-Profit Dementia Units (%)

	Nonprofit Homes (N = 15)	For-Profit Homes (N = 15)
Largely in-house transfers	46.7	33.3
Significant outside admissions	53.3	66.7

Notes: $p = 0.46$. Homes replying that 27% or fewer of their dementia unit admissions came from within their facility were redefined into the group with most admissions from the outside.

tically significant. In terms of facility size, 41.2 percent of smaller homes (those with a total bed capacity of 150 or fewer beds) admitted mostly from within the facility, compared with 38.5 percent of larger homes. Table 6.3 lists the figures regarding in-house transfers by facility size. Again the differences were not statistically significant. Thus, no significant differences were noted in the practice of admitting from within the facility in terms of either ownership status or facility size. Likewise, ownership status and facility size did not seem to influence a unit's likelihood of recruiting admissions from outside.

Administrators of dementia units were also asked if residents were grouped by either physical requirements or mental status. Such grouping did not seem to occur very often. Only 27.6 percent of the homes grouped dementia unit residents by physical requirements, and only 31 percent grouped residents by mental status. Thus, little subdivision of residents was being done. Perhaps this practice will occur more often in the future as providers become more comfortable with designating levels of care within units.

TABLE 6.3 Origin of Admissions to Dementia Units of Large and Small Homes (%)

	Large Homes (N = 13)	Small Homes (N = 17)
Largely in-house transfers	38.5	41.2
Significant outside admissions	61.5	58.8

Note: $p = 0.88$.

TABLE 6.4 Reported Frequency of Admitting Residents with the Goal of Discharging Them to a Lower Level of Care (%)

	Dementia Units (N = 30)	Comparison Units (N = 32)
Low frequency	93.3	75.0
High frequency	6.7	25.0

Notes: $p = 0.05$. Units responding "never" or "occasionally" were redefined into a low-frequency category; units responding "often" and "always" were redefined into a high-frequency category.

When asked about discharging residents to a lower level of care, available responses included "never," "occasionally," "often," and "always." "Never" and "occasionally" were redefined into a low-probability response, and "often" and "always" into a high-probability response. Nearly all (or 93.3 percent) of the dementia units fell in the low-probability group, whereas 75 percent of the comparison units did so. This difference was statistically significant ($p = .05$), indicating that the dementia units more often did not admit residents with the goal of transferring them to a lower level of care (see table 6.4).

Thus, our comparison units tended to be slightly more "rehabilitative" in outlook than the dementia units, which generally saw themselves as providing long-term care. We believe two explanations exist for these findings. First, the comparison units contained people with nondementia diagnoses, such as chronic pulmonary disease, stroke, or amputations. The units' "rehabilitative" philosophy reflected this different population, not a more favorable outlook toward dementia. Secondly, the fact that dementia units rarely set such high functional improvement goals represents a realistic appraisal of the rehabilitative potential of most dementia residents of nursing homes. Notable exceptions are: misdiagnoses (usually delirium diagnosed as dementia); respite care (a number of units provided respite services for families); and coexisting treatable diagnoses such as depression or hypothyroidism.

Further illustrating this point, administrators were also asked for the number of residents actually discharged to a lower level of care within the past 12 months. Dementia units had a mean rate of 2.1 residents moved to a lower level of care and a range of 0 to 9. Comparison units had a mean discharge rate of 18.7 and a range of 0 to 200. The differences were statistically significant ($p = .02$).

Last, in terms of admissions, dementia units were asked whether they specifically encouraged or discouraged residents with certain types of problems. Included were eight categories of behavioral and functional problems: confusion, wandering, agitation, verbal abuse, physical abuse, urinary incontinence, inability to ambulate, and feeding problems. The percentages of dementia units who encouraged, discouraged, or regarded indifferently admission of residents with these types of problems are listed in table 6.5. Dementia units more often encouraged admission of residents with confusion, wandering, and agitation. They most often discouraged residents who were physically abusive or nonambulatory. They tended to regard indifferently residents who were verbally abusive, had urinary incontinence, or had feeding problems.

Thus, the units we visited were attempting to work with demented residents with behavioral and functional problems commonly associated with the disease. However, like many long-term care settings, they limited certain types of behaviors, such as physical abusiveness. They also discouraged admission of nonambulatory people, perhaps reflecting the fact that these people were likely to be further along in the course of the illness and less able to benefit from specialized activities.

Ownership, Bed Capacity, Occupancy Rates, and Certification Levels

This section discusses other organizational characteristics of the facilities and the units. Facility-wide descriptions of ownership, size, and certification are summarized. Unit characteristics discussed are size, occupancy rates, and certification levels.

Table 6.6 displays our findings about facility characteristics. It includes characteristics of homes in our sample as well as comparative national data from the 1985 National Nursing Home Survey and the 1986 Inventory of Long-Term Care Places (Hing et al. 1989, Sirrocco 1989).

Because we intentionally drew approximately half of our sample from for-profit (proprietary) and half from nonprofit ownership status,

TABLE 6.5   Tendency to Admit Residents with Selected Problems (%)

	Dementia Units (N = 30)
Confusion	
Encouraged	93.3
Regarded indifferently	6.7
Discouraged	0.0
Wandering	
Encouraged	86.7
Regarded indifferently	13.3
Discouraged	0.0
Agitation	
Encouraged	53.3
Regarded indifferently	40.0
Discouraged	6.7
Verbal abusiveness	
Encouraged	26.7
Regarded indifferently	56.7
Discouraged	16.7
Physical abusiveness	
Encouraged	6.9
Regarded indifferently	34.5
Discouraged	58.6
Urinary incontinence	
Encouraged	30.0
Regarded indifferently	63.3
Discouraged	6.7
Nonambulatory status	
Encouraged	10.0
Regarded indifferently	26.7
Discouraged	63.3
Feeding problems	
Encouraged	16.7
Regarded indifferently	66.7
Discouraged	16.7

our sample was not representative of homes nationwide. In this country, about 75 percent of all homes are in the for-profit sector.

Dementia units in our sample tended to be found in large facilities. The average home with a dementia unit was about twice as large as the average nursing home in the United States. The average nursing home in this country has about 91.8 beds; our sample of dementia unit homes had an average of 190.6 beds.

When asked about bed certification in their facilities, administrators

TABLE 6.6 Ownership Status, Size, and Bed Certification of Facilities

	Study Sample		All U.S. Nursing Homes NNHS Data ($N = 19,100$)
	Dementia Units ($N = 30$)	Comparison Units ($N = 32$)	
Proprietary (%)	52[a]	56[a]	75[b]
Nonprofit (%)	48[a]	44[a]	25[b]
Mean no. of beds	190.6[c]	182.9[c]	91.8[d]
Medicare certification (%)	60[c]	71.9[c]	37[b]
Certified by Medicaid as SNF[e] (%)	60[c]	75[c]	41[b]
Certified by Medicaid as ICF[e] (%)	70[c]	75[c]	57[b]

[a]Our telephone survey of all five states found 61% of dementia units in proprietary homes and 39% in nonprofit homes. The study sample was not representative because we intentially selected about 50% in each ownership category.
[b]Source: Hing et al., 1989.
[c]Source: Study sample of 31 dementia units in five states.
[d]Source: Sirrocco (1989).
[e]SNF, skilled nursing facility; ICF, intermediate care facility.

answered in the following manner. About 60 percent of the dementia unit homes and 71.9 percent of the comparison unit homes were certified under Medicare. For those answering in the affirmative, the mean number of beds certified under Medicare was 75.9 for the dementia unit homes and 116.3 for the comparison unit homes. Considering the mean total number of beds in all facilities, this represented a majority of the beds in both settings, but higher totals in the comparison unit homes.

The likelihood of having Medicaid certification was also different for the settings. About 60 percent of the dementia unit homes and 75 percent of the comparison unit homes were certified under Medicaid as skilled nursing facilities (SNFs). For those facilities certified as SNFs, the mean number of beds certified was 95 for the dementia unit homes and 115.4 for the comparison unit homes.

There were similar findings for the facilities with regard to Medicaid certification as intermediate care facilities (ICFs). About 70 percent of the dementia unit homes and 75 percent of the comparison unit homes were certified under Medicaid as ICFs. For those facilities certified as ICFs, the mean number of beds certified was 71.7 for the dementia unit homes and 64.1 for the comparison unit homes. When contrasted with homes nationwide, our samples of both dementia unit and comparison unit homes tended to have more beds certified by Medicare and Medicaid.

In summary, the comparison unit homes had a higher percentage of their beds certified by Medicare and Medicaid, both as ICFs and SNFs. However, both the dementia unit and the comparison unit homes had higher percentages of their beds certified by Medicare and Medicaid when compared with homes nationwide. Another difference noted was that even though most facilities had the capacity to accept many Medicaid recipients, homes with dementia units tended to have an overall lower number of residents dependent on Medicaid reimbursement and a higher number of residents paying privately. This issue is discussed further in chapter 7.

In regard to the units themselves, dementia units were smaller than their nonspecialized counterparts. The mean bed capacity of dementia units studied was 35.9, with a range of 9 to 95 beds. The mean bed capacity on the comparison units was 59.1, with a range of 32 to 120 beds. This difference was statistically significant ($p < .001$).

Occupancy rates also differed between settings. Dementia units had a mean occupancy rate of 92 percent with a range of 67 to 100 percent. The comparison units had a mean occupancy rate of 97 percent, with a range of 84 to 100 percent. These differences were statistically significant ($p = .03$). Possible explanations for the slightly higher occupancy rates of comparison units include the newness of many dementia units and the likelihood that specialized units are more selective in their admissions.

The certification level of the units we visited did not differ much; this was a direct result of our attempts to match the settings one for one. Specifically, 50 percent of the dementia units and 46.9 percent of the comparison units were certified at the ICF level. A smaller number (36.7 percent of dementia units and 43.7 percent of comparison units) were certified at the SNF level. An even smaller percentage (13.3 percent of dementia units and 9.4 percent of comparison units) had dual certification. We also saw similarities due to geographic location. For example, because most nursing homes in California are certified at the SNF level, all of our units in that state had SNF certification. The size, occupancy rate, and certification level of units in our study are summarized in table 6.7.

In conclusion, a number of basic organizational features distinguished the dementia units from our comparison units. Dementia units tended to be found in larger facilities. Comparison units had a higher percentage of beds certified by Medicare and Medicaid. Average unit size differed, with dementia units generally being smaller than comparison units. Dementia units carefully selected their participants, often by a process that included a face-to-face interview. Admission policies reflected a strong preference for ambulatory, nonphysically abusive, confused elderly. Finally, dementia units had slightly lower occupancy rates.

TABLE 6.7 Size, Occupancy Rate, and Certification Level of Units

	Dementia Units (N = 30)	Comparison Units (N = 32)	p
No. of beds			
Mean	35.9	59.1	<.001
Range	(9–95)	(32–120)	
Occupancy rate (%)			
Mean	92	97	.03
Range	(67–100)	(84–100)	
Unit certification level (%)			
Intermediate care facility	50	46.9	>.05
Skilled nursing facility	36.7	43.7	
Both	13.3	9.4	

Some of these differences clearly arise from a philosophy that limits unit census and selects people believed most likely to benefit from unit services. The reasons for targeting services and limiting the number of participants become more evident in the chapters that follow.

Other Administrative Policies

In an attempt to look for differences in policies between settings, we asked three additional questions. These included whether or not the homes had participated in some form of dementia research in the past, whether or not the homes provided community services in the form of educational programs, and whether or not the home was affiliated with a university or medical school for purposes of student teaching. These findings are listed in table 6.8.

Dementia units were more likely to offer community services. A majority (80 percent) offered educational programs; only 37.5 percent of the comparison units replied that they offered this service ($p = .001$).

A significant difference was also noted in regard to whether or not the homes had contributed to dementia research. A majority of the dementia units, or 66.7 percent, stated that this was the case, while only 16.1 percent of the comparison unit homes answered in the affirmative ($p < .01$).

No differences were apparent, however, in the question regarding affiliation with a teaching institution. About 56.7 percent of the dementia units and 50 percent of the comparison units answered yes to this item.

TABLE 6.8   Units Providing Community Services, Contributing to Dementia Research, and Affiliated with a University (%)

	Dementia Units (N = 30)	Comparison Units (N = 32)	p
Provided community services			
Yes	80.0	37.5	<.001
No	20.0	62.5	
Contributed to research			
Yes	66.7	16.1	<.01
No	33.3	83.9	
Affiliated with a university			
Yes	56.7	50.0	.559
No	43.3	50.0	

Perhaps because the facilities were matched in several ways, an equal number in each category had characteristics similar to teaching nursing homes.

In summary, our dementia unit homes seemed more involved in dementia research and community educational programs about the disease. The existence of a specific unit serving this population of residents may have raised the level of awareness throughout the facility; this in turn may have distinguished the facilities with dementia units from most traditional nursing home settings.

Staffing Issues

In planning the study, conversations with experts in the field led us to believe that the staff providing care on these units was a key issue to address. This impression was reinforced by conversations with administrators. Some directors of units told us that if their resources were limited, their priority was always hiring qualified workers, as opposed to providing structural renovations. The specialized nature of these units meant that persons working there had to be carefully selected and trained to meet the demands of the setting. Consequently, we gathered data on three relevant staffing issues. These were the resident–staff ratio, the turnover rate for nursing staff, and a description of services provided for unit staff. Parallel data were collected on dementia and comparison units and are discussed in this section.

During our visits we noticed that many housekeeping staff members were attentive to the needs of the residents. While we did not specifically

TABLE 6.9 Mean Resident–Staff Ratios

	Dementia Units (N = 30)	Comparison Units (N = 32)
Licensed nursing staff	20.07:1	29.22:1
Nursing assistants	8.5:1	11.21:1
All nursing staff	5.97:1	8.1:1
Activities staff	50.6:1	84:1
Social workers	58.79:1	105.26:1

record their level of participation, we observed that they often spoke with residents and assumed a protective role. Some units had carefully chosen these workers, in view of their expected contact with the residents, and had included them in weekly interdisciplinary rounds. We acknowledge their importance, although we do not specifically report on their activities here.

RATIO OF RESIDENTS TO STAFF

The data on staffing ratios are discussed according to two formats. Because it is more commonly referred to, we begin by discussing the resident–staff ratio. This is given for each type of worker. Then we present our staffing data in terms of the number of staff hours per resident per week, which is more commonly used by administrators to figure actual costs of personnel.

Resident–staff ratios are listed in table 6.9. These figures are calculated for the period of a work week; or a total of 168 hours for the nursing staff, since coverage is required on a 24-hour basis. However, for activities staff, a work week is 84 hours, approximately 12 hours per day, seven days a week. For social workers, the ratio is expressed as full-time personnel per resident over a 40-hour week.

Licensed nursing staff includes registered nurses and licensed practical or vocational nurses. The ratio for this category of worker was 20.07 residents to 1 worker for the dementia units and 29.22 to 1 for the comparison units. The ratio for nursing assistants was 8.50 residents to 1 worker for the dementia units and 11.21 to 1 for the comparison units. For all nursing staff, the ratio was 5.97 residents to 1 staff member for the dementia units and 8.10 to 1 for the comparison units. Thus dementia units clearly staffed at a higher rate, or lower resident–staff ratio, than the comparison units in terms of nursing (see table 6.9).

Differences were also noted in activities staff and social workers.

TABLE 6.10 Staff Hours per Resident per Week

	Dementia Units	Comparison Units	p
Licensed nursing staff			
Mean	8.37	5.75	.015
Median	7.0	5.45	
Range	2.95–24.88	2.68–12.96	
Nursing assistants			
Mean	19.77	14.99	.075
Median	17.15	14.09	
Range	11–82	6.7–38.56	
All nursing staff			
Mean	28.15	20.74	.032
Median	24.29	19.61	
Range	15–104.96	10.38–51.52	
Activities staff			
Mean	1.66	1.0	.014
Median	1.68	0.71	
Range	0–4.44	0–3.33	
Social workers			
Mean	0.73	0.38	.04
Median	0.45	0.33	
Range	0–2.85	0–1.6	
All caregiver staff			
Mean	30.53	22.12	.02
Median	26.48	20.8	
Range	18.30–110.96	10.75–54.72	

Activities staff included the activities director and any activity aides. The ratio of residents to activities staff was 50.06 residents to 1 staff member for the dementia units and 84.0 to 1 for the comparison units. The resident–social worker ratio was 58.79 to 1 for the dementia units and 105.26 to 1 for the comparison units. Thus, as they did with nursing personnel, the dementia units staffed at a higher rate (lower resident–staff ratio) for these other categories of workers as well.

Table 6.10 presents the same data as mean hours of staff time per resident per week. For licensed staff, a mean of 8.37 hours per resident per week was observed on the dementia units, compared with 5.75 on the comparison units. For nursing assistants, the figure was 19.77 hours per resident per week for the dementia units and 14.99 for the comparison units. Figures for other categories of workers listed in table 6.10 also demonstrate differences between settings, with dementia units continuing to staff at higher rates (lower resident–staff ratios). The medians and ranges are provided to illustrate these differences further. The wide ranges for the dementia units indicate that a few of our units were staffing at a very high level.

Thus, the dementia units in our sample were providing a lower resident–staff ratio in every caregiver category. For every worker category, except the nursing assistants (where the differences approached significance), statistically significant differences were seen. The consistency of these findings suggests that dementia units believe higher staffing levels (lower resident–staff ratios) benefit the population they serve.

TURNOVER RATES FOR NURSING STAFF

The nursing staff of any facility is a group of workers whose presence is always required. This may lead to increased levels of stress and burnout in dementia units (Wilson and Patterson 1988). At times, stress results in high staff turnover, leading to care problems from new or temporary staff who are not familiar with residents.

Because of this, we were interested in studying staff turnover in the two settings. We asked administrators to provide us with an average yearly turnover rate for registered nurses, licensed practical nurses, and nursing assistants on their unit. Yearly turnover rate was defined as the percentage of workers who actually quit work during the previous year. That is, if 2 out of a total of 10 nursing assistants had left a unit, a 20 percent turnover rate was assigned to the unit for that category of worker. Because of the range of our findings in turnover rates, four levels were redefined. Units could either have 0 percent turnover, a 1 to 25 percent turnover, a 26 to 50 percent turnover, or over 50 percent turnover.

Tables 6.11, 6.12, and 6.13 display turnover rates for registered nurses, licensed practical nurses, and nursing assistants in the two settings. For registered nurses and for licensed practical nurses, the turnover rates in dementia units were lower than in comparison units. This difference was statistically significant for both registered nurses ($p = .003$) and licensed practical nurses ($p = .018$).

There was also a trend for nursing assistant turnover rates to be lower in dementia units, but this difference was not statistically significant ($p = .144$). It seemed that nursing assistants, in comparison to licensed staff, had turnover rates that were less different from the rates observed on comparison units. This may reflect the fact that, relative to comparison units, dementia units staffed higher in terms of licensed staff than nursing assistants.

During one of our site visits, an administrator told us that "burnout is another name for lack of administrative support." Our site visits documented unusual support for dementia unit staff through a variety of

TABLE 6.11   Average Turnover of Registered Nurses (%)

Turnover	Dementia Units (N = 27)	Comparison Units (N = 31)
0	63.0	25.8
1–25	14.8	48.4
26–50	3.7	19.3
>50	18.5	6.5

Note: $p = .003$.

TABLE 6.12   Average Turnover of Licensed Practical Nurses (%)

Turnover	Dementia Units (N = 28)	Comparison Units (N = 32)
0	39.3	18.8
1–25	21.4	56.2
26–50	28.6	9.4
>50	10.7	15.6

Note: $p = .018$.

TABLE 6.13   Average Turnover of Nursing Assistants (%)

Turnover	Dementia Units (N = 28)	Comparison Units (N = 32)
0	10.7	3.1
1–25	25.0	43.8
26–50	42.9	21.9
>50	21.4	31.2

Note: $p = .144$.

TABLE 6.14   Units Providing Services for Staff (%)

	Dementia Units (N = 30)	Comparison Units (N = 31)
Some staff services	76.7	70.9
No services	23.3	29.1

Note: $p = .61$.

mechanisms: (1) interest and concern in the unit itself on the part of facility administrators, sometimes to the extent that other areas of the facility did not feel as "special"; (2) more favorable resident–staff ratios; and (3) regular educational or problem-solving sessions for staff. Our data on turnover rates support the conclusion that burnout is not a greater problem on dementia units than elsewhere, probably in large measure because of the three supportive activities noted above.

SERVICES PROVIDED FOR STAFF

In keeping with the possibility of added stress for staff of dementia units, we attempted to assess whether these units were providing any services to alleviate this problem. In particular, we asked administrators if they offered staff support groups or gave them the option of rotating off the unit periodically to avoid burnout. In addition to these two forms of support, other services were reported. These included activities such as Alcoholics Anonymous groups, annual staff talent shows, baseball teams, and staff credentialing.

About 76.7 percent of the dementia units and 70.9 percent of the comparison units offered some type of staff support. These figures are listed in table 6.14; the differences did not reach statistical significance ($p = .61$), indicating that the dementia units did not differ from comparison units in their outlook on providing staff support. A high percentage of both types of settings we visited were offering some type of support for their workers. While the level was slightly higher on the dementia units, the difference was not statistically significant.

Conclusion

We conclude that the dementia units clearly differed in terms of certain staffing issues. Ratios of residents to staff were lower when compared to ratios for the traditional settings. This probably reflects a philosophy of providing more individualized care in a unique setting. It may also reflect the finding that dementia units tended to be found in larger homes possibly with more resources. The critical factor enabling dementia units to provide increased staff in comparison to traditional nursing home settings appears to be higher private pay revenues, as is discussed in chapter 7. Turnover rates were lower in dementia units for licensed staff but not for nursing assistants, possibly because the larger staff on dementia units did not have as much significance for nursing assistants. Staff support services were offered in both settings, and at only a slightly higher rate in the dementia units.

References

Hing, E. 1987. *Use of Nursing Homes by the Elderly. Preliminary Data from the National Nursing Home Survey.* National Center for Health Statistics. DHHS publication no. 87–1250. Public Health Service, Hyattsville, Md., May 14.

Hing, E., Sekscenski, E., and Strahan, G. 1989. *The National Nursing Home Survey: 1985 Summary for the United States.* National Center for Health Statistics. Series 13, No. 97. DHHS publication no. 89–1758. Public Health Service, Washington, D.C.: U.S. Government Printing Office.

Sirrocco, A. 1989. Nursing home characteristics: 1986 Inventory of long-term care places. National Center for Health Statistics. *Vital Health Statistics* 14(33).

Weiner, A. S., and Reingold, J. 1989. Special care units for dementia: Current practice models. *Journal of Long-Term Care Administration,* Spring, 14–19.

Wilson, R. W., and Patterson, M. A. 1988. Perceptions of stress among personnel on dementia units. *American Journal of Alzheimer's Care and Research* 3: 34–39.

7

Financial Considerations

PHILIP D. SLOANE, LAURA J. MATHEW,
AND WILLIAM G. WEISSERT

Dementia units, like other services in nursing homes, operate within a system where financial pressures are often great. Budgetary constraints are a fact of life for any nursing home, whether nonprofit or proprietary (for profit). All units must work diligently to cover operating expenses, the largest of which is personnel.

The current reimbursement system keeps nursing homes relatively full but tightly controls their revenues. Most nursing homes have a guaranteed clientele because regulatory processes limit the licensing of new homes. Because the majority of nursing home residents are financially destitute, however, their daily care is paid by Medicaid. By regulating the number of beds licensed, the states limit Medicaid costs and help existing homes operate at near capacity. In most states, however, Medicaid reimbursement rates are considered too low to assure the highest quality nursing home care possible.

To augment their revenues, homes attempt to attract private pay residents, whom they can charge a higher daily rate. These additional revenues allow the homes to provide additional staffing and services, as well as to increase their profit margin.

In this environment, new program initiatives, such as dementia units, must be evaluated in terms of their financial costs and benefits. If costs exceed the norm, then a program's continuation often rests on its ability to generate additional revenue for the facility, usually by attracting families that are willing to pay (privately) at higher rates.

Thus, the financial balance sheet is important in evaluating dementia units. In this chapter we report what we learned about the financial costs and revenues of the dementia units we visited. These data are limited, however, because financial questions were not the main emphasis of our study.

Costs of Care on Dementia Units

Proponents of dementia care often argue that optimal care requires more resource expenditure than traditional nursing home care. Among the purported cost increases are those due to environmental modifications and those that arise from increased staffing and programming. Our study data support the conclusion that dementia units generate additional costs.

ENVIRONMENTAL MODIFICATIONS

The features recommended for dementia units often require additional space, specialized construction, or special equipment. For example, wandering circuits, outdoor areas, alarm systems, and additional activity space all require larger initial outlays than do traditional nursing home settings.

One-fifth of the dementia units we visited had been especially constructed for dementia residents. An additional three-fifths had been renovated during or after conversion into specialized units. Table 7.1 summarizes these findings.

PROPORTION OF PRIVATE AND SEMIPRIVATE ROOMS

Another potential source of increased costs is the higher proportion of private rooms on dementia units. Our data indicate that dementia units have 22 percent of their bed capacity as private rooms, as opposed to 13 percent for the comparison units. As noted in table 10.2, this difference is statistically significant ($p < .001$).

From our discussions with nursing personnel, there seems to be a consensus that most dementia residents guard their own personal space and prefer a private room. Roommate disagreements are common. However, private rooms are often not built because they are more costly; they occupy more floor space and imply additional bathrooms. Thus, fewer private rooms exist in most units than would be ideal.

TABLE 7.1   Frequency of Renovations and New Construction

Extent of Building or Renovation	Units (%)
Especially constructed as a dementia unit	21
Structure renovated for the needs of a dementia unit	59
No renovations made	21

NURSING CARE NEEDS

By far the largest single expense of nursing home care is personnel, particularly the cost of nursing services. Our study classified all subjects into Resource Utilization Groups (RUGs) categories (see table 4.7). (RUGs is also known as the RUG-II instrument). Using these categories, we estimated nursing time requirements on the basis of estimates derived from studies of the RUGs in New York and Texas.

We calculated these figures using the RUGs classification system. The RUGs categorizes nursing home residents in 16 groups, each of which contains people whose nursing care needs are similar. These groups fall into the following categories: (1) special care residents, who have treatment or equipment requiring intensive nursing services, such as a respirator; (2) the rehabilitation group, which receives physical or occupational therapy at least five times weekly in an active rehabilitation program; (3) clinically complex residents who require active monitoring, usually because of a medical problem that is unstable (such as a poorly controlled seizure disorder) or requires a great deal of nursing time (such as a deep decubitus ulcer); (4) residents in the severe behavioral category, who currently demonstrate behavioral problems so disruptive (e.g., physical aggressiveness or feces smearing) that they interfere markedly with care and often with life on the unit; and (5) the physical categories, which include residents receiving custodial care because of impaired activities of daily living (ADLs) who do not fit into any of the other categories. Within each of the above five categories are subgroups based on the degree of ADL impairment.

Table 7.2 lists the percentage of subjects in each RUGs category among subjects in the dementia units and comparison units we studied. The table also includes estimates of how much nursing time each category of resident requires, based on data gathered during field tests of the RUGs system in New York and Texas. These estimates were used to compute and compare the amount of nursing time required by dementia unit and comparison unit residents.

From table 7.2, one can see that the comparison units had higher

TABLE 7.2   Case Mix Patterns and Estimated Nursing Staff Needs

RUG-II Category	Nursing Time per Resident		Residents	
			In Dementia Units (N = 303)	In Comparison Units (N = 317)
	New York	Texas		
	mean minutes/day		%	
1. Special care A	246.6	124.0	0	0
2. Special care B	279.0	157.0	1.32	2.84
3. Rehabilitation A	154.2	120.0	0	0
4. Rehabilitation B	208.0	117.0	0	1.26
5. Clinically complex A	117.0	72.5	0.66	0.32
6. Clinically complex B	198.6	108.1	0.33	1.26
7. Clinically complex C	229.8	123.2	1.65	2.21
8. Clinically complex D	286.2	130.9	0	2.52
9. Severe behavioral A	119.4	47.1	2.97	2.84
10. Severe behavioral B	180.0	90.0	17.16	9.46
11. Severe behavioral C	229.8	131.4	3.96	6.31
12. Physical A	93.0	42.1	18.15	11.99
13. Physical B	144.6	78.4	10.89	2.52
14. Physical C	179.4	91.8	26.07	30.91
15. Physical D	213.0	115.1	7.26	10.41
16. Physical E	259.8	127.6	9.57	15.14

Estimated nursing care minutes per day needed per 100 residents:

Based on New York estimates			17,216	19,240
Based on Texas estimates			8,766	9,867

Note: All nursing staff. Unpublished data courtesy of Brant Fries, Ph.D., University of Michigan.

proportions of individuals in the heaviest care categories. Particularly noteworthy is the high proportion of comparison unit subjects in the physical D and physical E groups. In contrast, dementia units contained more individuals in the severe behavioral groups and in the less impaired physical A and physical B groups.

These results showed that comparison unit residents require more nursing care than dementia unit residents. In other words, the case mix of the comparison units appears to include more heavy-care residents than that of the dementia units, implying the need for more nursing services.

To quantify the extent of these case mix differences, we estimated nursing requirements per 100 residents for the dementia units and comparison units. These estimates are noted at the bottom of table 7.2. The estimated hours based on New York and Texas data were quite different (suggesting a remarkable variation in expectations of care between the two states), but the ratio of estimated care needs between comparison units and dementia units was almost identical: 1.118 using New York data and 1.126 using Texas data. Thus, comparison unit residents are estimated on average to require a little more than 10 percent more nursing time than dementia unit residents. The mean of these figures (1.122) is used in the next section to adjust resident–staff ratios for case mix.

STAFFING LEVELS

Chapter 6 presented data indicating that resident–staff ratios are lower on dementia units than comparison units. Table 6.9 summarized these results. It indicates that dementia units on average employed more staff per resident than did the comparison units. These differences were statistically significant for licensed nursing staff, all nursing staff, activities staff, social workers, and all caregiver staff. The difference in nursing assistant staffing did not quite achieve statistical significance, but since it demonstrates a trend in the same direction, it is consistent with the other categories.

Correction for Case Mix Differences

Since our comparison units managed more residents requiring heavy care than did the dementia units, we attempted to adjust for this case mix difference using the figure calculated from the RUGs scores in table 7.2. In table 7.3 we apply this case mix correction to the resident–staff ratio for all nursing staff. The median ratio, rather than the mean, was used for these calculations to mitigate the effect of a couple of dementia units that were outliers (and staffed much higher than other units). If our assumptions are correct (that the RUGs scores estimate care needs of the subjects studied, and that within each unit studied our study subjects are representative of all residents), then dementia units provide approximately 1.4 hours of nursing services per resident for every hour of services per resident provided by the comparison units.

Proprietary versus Nonprofit Units

Next, we studied for-profit and nonprofit dementia units separately to determine if their staffing levels were different. No statistically significant differences were present for any of the staffing categories (licensed nursing staff, nursing assistants, all nursing staff, activities personnel, social workers, and all staff).

TABLE 7.3   Relative Staffing of Dementia Units versus Comparison Units

$$\text{Staffing ratio} = \frac{\text{Hours/resident/week}_{\text{dementia}}{}^{\text{a}}}{\text{Hours/resident/week}_{\text{comparison}}{}^{\text{a}}} \times \text{Case mix correction}^{\text{b}}$$

$$= \frac{24.29}{19.61} \times 1.12 = 1.39 \text{ nursing staff (licensed nurses or nursing assistants) employed by dementia units for each nursing employee of comparison units}$$

[a]Median statistics used.

[b]Case mix correction = $\dfrac{\begin{array}{l}\text{Estimated minutes per day of nursing time needed}\\ \text{by comparison unit residents (from RUG)}\end{array}}{\begin{array}{l}\text{Estimated minutes of nursing time needed by}\\ \text{dementia unit residents (from RUG)}\end{array}}$

$= 1.122$

Conclusion

Dementia units appear to staff higher than the comparison units. Adjusting for case mix, the units studied appear to staff at a level more than a third higher than comparison units. No difference is apparent in staffing levels between for-profit and nonprofit units.

Reimbursement Issues

Having demonstrated costs to be higher on dementia units, we now look at the other side of the balance sheet, reimbursement. As was noted in the introduction to this chapter, private pay revenues provide an important support for the increased costs incurred by a dementia unit. Therefore, the first consideration is to compare the proportion of private pay residents in dementia units to that in comparison units.

Payment source data from the 307 dementia unit and 318 comparison units residents we studied indicate that dementia units contain a higher proportion of private residents. On average, nearly 60 percent of dementia unit residents paid privately, compared with about 33 percent of comparison unit residents. These figures were nearly identical for both nonprofit and proprietary facilities (see table 7.4).

Charges and reimbursement rates among the facilities we studied are summarized in table 7.5, which shows that 79 percent of nursing homes with dementia units charged private residents more for the dementia unit than they did for other nursing units at the same certification level. That excess charge varied from unit to unit and from state to state.

TABLE 7.4   Primary Payment Source of Residents (%)

	In Dementia Units (N = 307)	In Comparison Units (N = 318)
All facilities*		
Third-party payers (primarily Medicaid)	41.4	67.0
Private pay	58.6	33.0
Nonprofit facilities**		
Third-party payers (primarily Medicaid)	39.5	63.1
Private pay	60.5	36.9
For-profit facilities**		
Third-party payers (primarily Medicaid)	42.0	69.7
Private pay	58.0	30.3

*Chi-square$_1$ = 41.3, $p < .001$.
**Mantel-Haenszel chi-square = 41.1, $p < .001$.

In all cases, private pay room rates exceeded Medicaid reimbursement rates. The average amount of this difference ranged between 16 percent for Ohio intermediate care facilities (ICFs) and 162 percent for California skilled nursing facilities (SNFs). No Medicaid provider reimbursed a nursing home in our study more for dementia unit care than for care at other nursing units at the same certification level.

Conclusion

Dementia units appear to provide services that are more costly than traditional nursing home services for residents with Alzheimer's disease and related disorders. They often are especially constructed, or are renovated for use, as specialized units. They staff higher in all direct care personnel, including licensed nursing staff, nursing assistants, activities personnel, and social workers.

These additional costs are largely recovered through private payers. The proportion of private residents is considerably higher on dementia units than in our comparison units. In addition, most nursing homes with dementia units charge higher private rates for dementia unit care than for care in other nursing areas at the same certification level.

TABLE 7.5 Private Pay Charges of Dementia Units

State	Certification Level[a]	Cost Differential between Dementia Unit and Other Units[b] No	Cost Differential between Dementia Unit and Other Units[b] Yes	Mean Excess Charge of Dementia Unit	For Units Accepting Medicaid[c] Mean Private Pay Rate	For Units Accepting Medicaid[c] Mean Medicaid Rate[d]
California	SNF	1	4	$19.75	$122.50	$46.76
North Carolina	ICF	2	4	8.50	67.30	48.20
	SNF	1	—	—	108.00	66.34
New York	HRF	0	2	18.00	92.80	55.70
	SNF	0	4	16.00	183.20	129.70
Ohio	ICF	1	3	3.17	54.50	47.00
	SNF	0	2	8.75	82.00	58.90
Texas	ICF	1	3	5.67	50.00	35.13

Note: This information is based on data collected between November 1987 and February 1989.
[a]SNF, skilled nursing facility; ICF, intermediate care facility; HRF, health-related facility.
[b]Three units were excluded from this table: one California and one Texas facility had no other units at the same level of care as the dementia unit; one Texas facility failed to complete the administrative questionnaire.
[c]One unit in California, two in Texas, one in North Carolina, and two in Ohio did not accept Medicaid.
[d]None of the facilities studied received differential Medicaid reimbursement for dementia units compared with other units certified at the same level of care.

Discussion

These results are consistent with expectations in some respects. Dementia units attract more private pay residents, charge more, and staff more heavily. However, the results are counterintuitive in one important respect: dementia unit residents appear to require less care than those on comparison units. What makes this surprising is that one motivation for creating dementia units is to put dementia residents in a setting where they can receive more care. Several possible explanations for these findings arise.

One possibility is that the RUGs classification system is not capturing all the care needs of dementia residents. This remains an area of debate in the field of long-term care reimbursement. RUG-II differs from earlier versions of this classification scheme precisely in its treatment of dementia. It was modified specifically to capture care needs associated with dementia-related behavioral problems that were being missed by earlier measurement tools. Effects of dementia on staff time provided to residents were measured in time and motion studies to produce the new version. Its author (Foley 1986) claims that

> the system . . . is far from insensitive to the needs of dementia residents who require supervision or intervention and do not demonstrate behavioral problems. The RUGs system, through use of the Activities of Daily Living index, provides an extremely refined means to measure the level of assistance required for the exact types of activities mentioned. Those residents who require constant supervision can be discriminated from those requiring intermittent supervision or assistance.

Assuming that the RUGs designers are correct, the explanation for our finding that less care is needed by dementia residents but more care capability is available on dementia units must lie elsewhere.

The most likely explanation is market pressures that require nursing homes to compete for both private pay residents and nursing staff. Often the motivation for offering a dementia unit is to attract more private pay residents. Homes compete by offering features intended to attract and keep the most profitable residents—those who can pay privately.

We compared the degree of competition for private pay residents (measured as the number of empty nursing home beds per 1,000 elderly residents) with the number of dementia units existing in our five study states and found a positive correlation of just under 50 percent. While this figure is not strong enough to justify the conclusion that competition is the only force driving the development of specialized units, the fact that dementia units appear to become more prevalent as the number of empty beds increases suggests that attempts at nonprice competition is a large part of the explanation.

Assuming that is the case, then it follows that homes offering dementia units may also use staffing levels to differentiate their home and to lure private pay residents. Family caregivers are likely to compare units on the basis of resident–staff ratios. Of course, extra staffing will cause costs to rise, but if consumers see no close substitutes, their demand for care will be relatively nonresponsive to price.

In addition to competing for private pay residents, homes have another incentive to generously staff their dementia units. That is, they must compete for scarce staff, especially professional nursing staff. Units that are generously staffed are likely to be most attractive to potential staff members and most successful in keeping existing staff.

Thus the dementia unit manager, trying to attract private pay residents and retain competent nursing personnel, staffs at lower than traditional resident–staff ratios. This in turn leads to prices above nondementia unit prices, as is consistent with our findings.

While the RUGs instrument suggests that dementia unit residents do not require more care than those on our comparison units, we would expect them to have access to more organized activities and to be cared for by specially trained staff engaging in activities that reflect special attention to the residents' unique needs. Again, our observations on resident care (see chapter 2) confirmed these expectations.

The question of the efficiency and effectiveness of the extra staff remains unanswered. Ideally, extra staff, extra activities, and more appropriate types of interactions with residents should produce better resident outcomes. On the other hand, such nonprice competition can potentially lead to increased costs without increased quality.

This study's findings on the quality of care (see chapters 2 and 4) are mixed and are limited by its cross-sectional nature. We found dementia unit residents to be more mobile, physically restrained less often, and more often involved in interactions with staff and other residents. On the other hand, chemical restraints and behavioral problems were not lower on dementia units. Controlled longitudinal studies would be required, however, to separate the effects of resident selection (and discharge) policies from the effects of the care provided.

Thus, we cannot yet determine the effects of increased staffing on dementia units. If process and outcome indicators of quality are indeed better on such units, then that raises a question of equity for non–private pay dementia residents. If no differences are found, then dementia units are unlikely to win administrative approval for extra staffing and extra reimbursement. Since RUGs shows less care required by dementia unit residents, a case could be built for extra payment only if better, and therefore more appropriate, outcomes can be demonstrated.

Finally, the rapid growth of dementia units suggests that the field may soon be saturated. According to estimates by Leon et al. (1989), as many as 14 percent of nursing homes nationally will operate such units. Over time, many homes in highly competitive areas will probably find that they cannot attract enough private pay residents to sustain extra staff on these units. As they cut staff, they will lose residents, until the number of homes with units stabilizes at a point where those that exist can operate efficiently and prices reflect efficient use of extra staff. This prospect suggests that some homes may want to consider whether in the long run they are likely to be losers or winners in the competition for private pay dementia residents. If their prognosis is to be long-run losers, they might want to avoid getting into the market, perhaps concentrating instead on fighting for other types of residents.

References

Foley, W. J. 1986. *Dementia among Nursing Home Patients: Defining the Condition, Characteristics of the Demented, and Dementia on the RUG-II Classification System.* Troy, N.Y.: Rensselaer Polytechnic Institute.

Leon, J., Potter, D. E. B., and Cunningham, P. J. 1990. Current and Projected Availability of Special Nursing Home Programs for Alzheimer's Disease Patients. DHHS publication no. 90–3463. National Medical Expenditure Survey Data Summary 1, Agency for Health Care Policy and Research. Rockville, Md.: Public Health Service.

8

Establishing a Dementia Unit

NANCY K. ORR-RAINEY

The decision to develop specialized Alzheimer's services in the nursing home should be made with careful consideration. A dementia unit can potentially have both a positive and a negative impact on the facility residents, staff, and community. It can come to be regarded as either one of the best or one of the worst decisions made by a nursing facility. The outcome depends, to a large measure, on just how much analysis and planning are done and the effort put into design and implementation.

Nursing home operators hope that by creating a dementia unit in their facility several positive things will happen. Most often providers hope that the service will help improve the care of a difficult population. Alzheimer's disease residents can be a liability for a facility. They wander frequently and are at risk for leaving the facility and getting lost. They can interfere with the care of other residents, sometimes to the point of jeopardizing health and safety. No provider or nursing staff wishes to use pharmacological or physical restraints unnecessarily, but lack of an appropriate physical plant and care management techniques may leave few other options. The suggestion to create a special environment, therefore, is often made first by nursing staff eager to find new ways to care for Alzheimer's disease residents.

Secondly, a provider may be interested in developing a dementia unit to attract more residents. There may be excessive competition in the area for nursing home care, and specialized services can help create a market niche. If the dementia unit is done well, the program also carries with it the added benefit of improving the resident mix. In other words, the overall percentage of private pay residents in the facility will increase.

A dementia unit in an established building can also create a number of positive internal effects. It can boost staff morale, attract new staff, and uplift the facility's overall image. In the best of situations it can improve the census in the rest of the facility because consumers begin to recognize the facility's leadership and innovation in the care of elderly people.

But there is also potential for a dementia unit to create more problems than it solves. Initiated without proper planning and market analysis, a program can become an inappropriate way of delivering resident care and a financial disaster. To avoid these and other problems it is critical to begin by assessing the feasibility of a dementia unit with a full market analysis. Assuming that the results are encouraging, the next steps demand conscientious planning and implementation.

The majority of what is discussed in this chapter is the result of eight years of pioneering, hands-on experience in program development. This chapter is not meant to provide a foolproof method of developing a dementia unit. Rather, it is meant to serve as a guide. There were no models to follow or other programs to learn from in 1982, when the Hillhaven Corporation in Tacoma, Washington, began developing dementia units (special care units). We were guided by a desire to do something different, something better, and something the company could be proud of. If your guiding principles are similar, you are unlikely to fail in your endeavors. Hillhaven has been largely successful with dementia units, growing and changing as we learn more. But we have also made some mistakes, stumbled, and fallen along the way. This chapter aspires to lend some insight and make the process easier and more successful for others.

Market Analysis

A detailed analysis of the potential market for a dementia unit does not have to be an intimidating, long-drawn-out process. A thorough job can be completed in one to three weeks, depending on the risks involved and the tasks that must be accomplished. All market analyses should include a review of internal and external factors affecting a facility.

INTERNAL FACTORS

Internal factors include what is happening inside the facility in which development of a dementia unit is being considered. First, find out why there is interest in the program. If the main reason is to attract residents, it is important to find out why a census problem exits. It may be that the service area is overbedded and competition intense. It may be that the facility has a poor reputation. If so, why? How well deserved is the reputation? What has been done to turn the situation around? It is a mistake to begin a program to solve a census problem without understanding the root cause and correcting it. Hillhaven learned early on in the development process that unless a facility with a past history of problems has a stable leadership and has clearly "turned the corner" in correcting problems, a dementia unit cannot provide the magic solution to poor census.

Another key element in internal evaluation has to do with physical plant. In most cases, providers adapt a physical plant that is already in existence. Hillhaven has established standards that must be met by dementia units. These include in-unit space for group activities and dining, the ability to segregate approximately 20 to 25 beds into a separate unit, and accessibility to outside areas. Evaluation should also include the amount, quality, and accessibility of space for supply storage (including soiled linens), staff charting, medication preparation, and resident bathing. Few nursing care centers considering a dementia unit have the luxury of designing exactly what they want and getting it all.

Adaptation should always consider resident needs as the first priority and staff needs secondarily. Decisions often come down to providing what the unit "must have" and compromising the "nice to have" category because of costs involved in reconstruction or construction.

Activity and dining spaces are absolutely critical, and they must accommodate everyone comfortably. Crowded common areas can create impossible care conditions. An outside courtyard further increases residents' common space and encourages therapeutic physical activity. If your internal analysis of the physical plant fails to turn up a way of providing these three critical elements, you should not continue with the feasibility study. However, few facilities cannot find a way to alter a physical plant. The hindrance is usually how much the facility is able to invest financially, not whether alteration is possible.

The greatest operational cost for program implementation usually involves a loss of beds to make available adequate common space for the unit residents. If land is available, the common space can be constructed. If the facility cannot build the common space, a lost bed means lost revenue. Unfortunately, state Medicaid systems do not recognize the benefit of common space when it comes to the care of Alzheimer's disease residents. No state Medicaid system will reimburse the cost of that lost bed. The provider must recapture that cost either in the rates set for the program or in the census gain. In some states, once a bed is taken out of circulation, the loss is permanent. You should know what the laws are before deciding to take beds out of circulation.

Refurbishment and addition of a security system cost money. In the best of situations the costs of these physical plant alterations are approximately $7,000. If new construction is necessary, costs as high as $200,000 may be incurred for a 25-bed unit.

The final area of internal analysis involves resident care. The facility's ability to staff properly should weigh heavily in the development decision. The consistent use of contract labor, both licensed and un-licensed, is a serious concern. High staff turnover, frequent staff changes, or rotation of staff in and out of a dementia unit can be disastrous because many residents of these units adjust to changes poorly. Therefore, decision makers should be relatively certain that the use of contract labor will not affect program operations. In some cases, when other key areas are strong and stable, a dementia unit can eliminate staff turnover and attract new staff desiring a challenge and a new opportunity to learn. This, however, is more the exception than the rule.

Finally, the current quality of care must be examined, but it is often difficult to judge objectively. Past or recent federal and state surveys are helpful but do not predict staff ability to learn or to make changes. Confidence in the nursing leadership is crucial and undoubtedly involves subjective and objective judgment. Eventually, staff education will make the difference in caregiving; adequate energy and resources must be dedicated to it. Staff issues are discussed in detail later in the chapter.

THE EXTERNAL REVIEW

An external review usually involves what most people consider when they think of marketing. Knowing the competition or lack of it has bearing on what you are able or willing to do. For example, if your service area is already overbedded and there are two or three other providers with dementia units, you will want to know what the competing units are like and how successful they are. This should involve visits to the competitors and discussions with other community service providers about how they perceive the services currently offered by your competitors. It is always desirable to be the first or only provider of a unique service, but this is increasingly difficult to do in the area of Alzheimer's care. For the first five years of Hillhaven's development we rarely had competition. Now it is the exception to be the first or sole provider in an area. Competition is healthy. It means that you must be capable of doing as good a job as, or better than, someone else and that you continue to do so after the program begins.

When a good deal of competition exists or significant financial risks are involved in developing a dementia unit, it is probably wise to obtain information on the demographics of the area. Advertising agencies or market research firms can quickly and reliably evaluate the market area for you. In particular, you will want to know the number of people over the age of 65 and apply the prevalence and incidence rates for Alzheimer's disease to this population. If you are concerned about the census mix of your population, then it is wise to cross-reference for income.

Just a few years ago some service providers believed that specialized dementia services might be so attractive that families would be willing to travel great distances to place a family member. This has not been the experience of the Hillhaven Corporation. Working in 23 states and operating more than 50 dementia units, we have found that families strongly prefer to place their relatives close to home so they can visit frequently and stay involved in care. This has been true even in states where only one dementia unit was available and was advertised heavily throughout a large geographical area. Our experience is that, regardless of how special the service is, families will rarely travel beyond a 20-mile radius for nursing home care.

Finally, the person with Alzheimer's disease is rarely the one who decides that nursing home care is needed. The children or spouse usually make this decision. Frequently, family members want to relocate an impaired relative for nursing home care near them. But demographic information on family members is much less reliable and more difficult to interpret than data on people with dementia. Information about family members might be better used in the actual marketing of your services rather than in determining whether or not a need exists in the first place.

One possible explanation for the sudden growth in specialized Alzheimer's care has been the confidence that there are plenty of residents to fill whatever empty beds may exist in a nursing home. Given rough figures on the number of people currently residing in nursing homes who suffer from some form of cognitive impairment, there is little doubt that specialized dementia services of some type would be of value. According to the 1987 National Nursing Home Survey, demented residents exceed 50 percent of nursing home residents. So unless the competition in the area is extremely tough, extensive demographic analysis is usually not necessary.

The question I am most frequently asked is "How did Hillhaven know what would work when they designed their dementia units?" The answer is that no substitute replaces talking with and working with Alzheimer's disease families. Whether you decide to conduct a formal focus group through a marketing and advertising agency or attend local support groups, families are eager to discuss what they want from nursing home care. Gathering information from families still caregiving at home is invaluable as you begin to decide on your capabilities for delivering services. One thing is certain: families will not buy average nursing home care. If the service is different (lacking in the heavy use of pharmacological and physical restraints, for example), then families will want to place their relatives in the program.

The provider must be prepared to be visibly different from the competition and address the service needs of the family consumer. While families usually affirm the need for specialized services (Yankelovich et al. 1986), they are not necessarily good at specifying what "special" means. Often families are not familiar with nursing home care, choosing not to think about it until placement time comes. This situation may be changing, however. The Alzheimer's Association's publication of a consumer guide for nursing home care and specialized services is one evidence of change. Increasingly, families are demanding more information about nursing home care, and their expectations reflect it. Continued research in this area is also likely to further consumer knowledge.

Evaluating community services that assist dementia patients and families is critical. Be careful, however, in interpreting the feedback providers give you. Occasionally, the community service professionals who provide day care, home health, and other dementia services strongly believe that their job is to keep patients out of nursing homes for as long as possible—even when this policy is detrimental to caregivers and patients. The only way to combat this attitude effectively is to include these providers in your planning process and reassure them of your intentions. The majority of service providers and especially the Alzheimer's Association chapters will welcome your involvement in the service network.

Talking to families and nonimpaired residents already in the nursing facility may provide you with some of the best ideas for developing your service. At the very least, your current consumers should not be overlooked. At best, you will remember to include them in all phases of your planning and implementation. This will help ward off potential jealousies if the program becomes a reality. It is important that everyone involved with the facility feel a part of the development process.

Once all the external information is gathered, it needs to be combined with the internal information and reviewed carefully. Rarely is any situation guaranteed success. In the majority of cases risks must be weighed, and weaknesses and strengths balanced. Then a decision is made.

Experience has taught Hillhaven that high levels of motivation in tackling a new program can overcome even the most difficult obstacles, but without that motivation and desire a program is almost certain to fail. Unless the administration and leadership of a building have the right attitude, no amount of market research will matter. An intense desire to be innovative and to provide high-quality care, however, will always prevail.

The Program Design

GOALS

The marketing information obtained from the internal and external evaluations should answer questions about whom you will be serving and what they will want. With that information, the nursing home leadership must choose the program's goals or "mission." To inspire staff with a sense of mission, clear, measurable strategies for obtaining it must be provided. These strategies will form the basis of program design.

Hillhaven designed its special care unit (SCU) programs to meet the needs of dementia residents who would present care problems in a more traditional area of the facility. This group is a subset of the dementia population because many residents never develop severe behavioral problems. As a rule of thumb, these residents are at risk for wandering, interfering with other residents' care, and exhibiting a wide variety of other behavioral problems such as hitting, biting, scratching, and disruptive vocalizations. Not long ago, most providers viewed these residents as "undesirable." Families had an extremely difficult time finding placement and when they did, the residency was often short lived.

The Hillhaven Corporation then chose a mission to reflect the needs of the population it decided to serve. The goal had to be simply stated and easily remembered by everyone: to deliver care without the use of chemical and physical restraints. This is what the company believes families want and expect from specialized Alzheimer's services. Keeping a mission simple is important because everyone involved needs to understand it and believe in it. But while Hillhaven's mission is stated simply, accomplishing it is a constant challenge. That is why well-thought-out strategies whose success can be measured are critical. In the long run, to accomplish a mission, you must relate every program component directly back to that mission. Otherwise people lose sight of what they are doing.

THE POPULATION TO BE SERVED

It is difficult to generalize, but most professionals in and outside the nursing home industry have come to believe that residents with severe behavioral problems are most likely to benefit from a specialized unit. This subset of the dementia population tends to have fewer skilled nursing needs or complicating medical problems than other nursing home residents. That is not to say that they are not at risk for complicated medical problems. In fact, dementia residents may be at greater risk because of their inability to report problems or to verbally register discomfort. This is why professional nursing care is necessary. For example, dementia residents are at significant risk for the inappropriate use of psychotropic medications. Often when residents are ill with treatable illnesses, such as urinary infections (UTIs), behavior worsens. They can become combative or perhaps refuse to eat. Since their cognitive impairment makes it difficult for them to report the discomfort associated with a UTI, their behavior problem may be treated with a psychotropic drug and the UTI ignored until it is advanced. Hillhaven's experience indicates that as many as a third of dementia unit residents come into the program with an unrecognized and untreated medical problem like cystitis, overmedication, or depression. Clearly, the medical, psychological, and social needs of the dementia resident need to be considered. A good program design will work to achieve balance among them.

Little to no information about specialized units for very advanced dementia residents is available, although the idea is worth considering. A few facilities, such as the Hebrew Home for the Aged in Riverdale, New York, and Heather Hill in Chardon, Ohio, have developed multiple units, one or more of which is for very advanced dementia residents. If you are interested in serving this population, and the need has been proven by your market analysis, hospice models may be helpful in designing a program. Hillhaven's experience, however, is that families are more likely to request nursing home care when behavioral problems are extreme— usually much earlier in the disease process.

If families can make it to the point where their relative is no longer ambulatory or combative, they have often made it through the most difficult time. The specialized dementia unit for difficult behavioral problems will, therefore, be of little help. Not all behavioral problems improve as Alzheimer's disease worsens, however. Noisiness is most prevalent among those who are dependent in all activities of daily living (Jackson et al. 1989). In addition, families often need nursing home care late in the disease, when medical needs become overwhelming. Such residents usually qualify for a Medicare-certified or skilled level of nursing home care. It might be a good idea to place special emphasis on the training of staff in these skilled areas to assure that their knowledge incorporates the needs of the dementia resident.

ADMISSION AND DISCHARGE CRITERIA

Whatever subgroup of the dementia population you choose to serve, admission and discharge criteria should be explicit. These criteria define the population served and help the nursing home do the best possible job

TABLE 8.1   Admission and Discharge Criteria for Hillhaven's
Special Care Units

Admission criteria (both must be met)

Family interview is completed.
  Complete psychosocial history
  Memory and behavior checklist
  Family burden interview
  Biographical sketch

Resident assessment confirms dementia and rules out delirium.
  Mental status exam
  DSM-III
  Blood chemistry screening

Discharge criteria (any one constitutes an indication for discharge)

Functional status is significantly reduced.
  Total loss of ambulation skills
  Total dependency in eating, dressing, and grooming
  Terminal care needed

A complex medical problem needs skilled care and outweighs the dementia.

A behavioral problem cannot be managed without the use of chemical or
physical restraints and causes danger to self or others, in spite of the best
efforts of unit staff and physicians.

The resident cannot participate in or receive benefit from group activities
whether because of
  One of the above situations
  Misdiagnosis or improvement in status (due to treatment of complicating
    factors)

---

of serving it. To care for a specific population requires an organized
strategy.

Admission criteria for a dementia unit can range from very formal to
extremely informal because there are no state or federal requirements.
Some programs make placement decisions on the basis of function. Others consider only diagnosis. Still others segregate residents solely on the
basis of their behavior (i.e., all noisy residents are put on the unit).

Hillhaven chose a formal preadmission screening process (table 8.1).
For the past five years we have worked to assure accuracy of diagnosis, to
identify and manage problems that are treatable, and to gather information that will assist in delivering high-quality resident care. Initially, we
operated without such criteria. Despite honest intentions, most of our
early programs had a mixed population of mentally ill and dementia
residents. From these experiences we learned that (1) assessment and
diagnosis are serious problems in some nursing homes and (2) relying

solely on the medical community for accurate diagnosis is foolish. A specialized dementia program must be prepared, therefore, to verify a diagnosis and rule out treatable causes of unusual, or what is often labeled "senile," behavior. Another reason for establishing admission criteria is that information gathered before a resident's arrival can have great bearing on adjustment to the new living arrangement. Residents admitted without information from families about how they actually function may not benefit from care on the unit.

Problems can often be avoided by informing staff about preferences or routines of a new resident. Preadmission assessment should include information about past and present function, including problems and circumstances affecting the resident's current functioning. Results from some of Hillhaven's preadmission assessments indicate that a large percentage of families report significant changes in functioning in the few months preceding placement. Often this is due to treatable factors that should be addressed either before or immediately after placement on the dementia unit.

For example, to find that a family and their impaired relative have been through two changes in living environment, several different trials of medication to control behavior, and a recent hospitalization is not unusual. Few families understand that increased behavioral problems are associated with relocation trauma. It is the staff's responsibility not only to explain what may be happening but also to help the family and resident through difficulties until behavior improves. In some cases the end result may be that the resident's behavior improves and the family decides that placement is no longer needed.

A good example can be seen in an admission to one of our dementia units in California. A woman had been caring for her husband at home for a number of years. As his disease progressed, his behavior worsened. He became easily upset, yelling at his wife and accusing her of stealing his money. He would often pace throughout the house for hours and would awaken at night threatening to leave. Emotionally upset and physically drained from lack of sleep, the woman first sought help from her physician. He prescribed haloperidol, but the behavior worsened. The woman then tried day care so that she could get some rest, but the day care program was unable to manage her husband.

Suffering from the effects of haloperidol and other medications, the patient sustained a fall and broke his hip. He was hospitalized, and surgery was performed. By the time he entered our facility, he was completely nonambulatory. He had received no physical therapy because of his cognitive and behavioral problems. His medications had been increased in an attempt to control his behavior in the hospital. He could not communicate or feed, bathe, or dress himself. He had a Foley catheter to deal with his incontinence. Dementia unit staff viewed this resident as a good candidate for rehabilitation and restorative care. Physical therapy, which was covered by Medicare, was prescribed, and he was soon walking again. As his psychotropic medication was reduced, the resident began to feed himself again and to regain the 20 pounds he had lost. The Foley catheter was discontinued, and he was placed on a bowel and bladder training program. Thus, the resident went from being totally dependent in all activities of daily living to needing minimal assistance.

In the meantime his wife was getting the much needed rest that she deserved. Eventually her involvement in the local support group helped her understand and cope with her husband's behavior. By talking with staff and the dementia unit's medical consultant she reached an understanding of her husband's condition. She decided to take him back home and to use home care and day care again before deciding on final placement.

The dementia unit staff facilitated this gradual rehabilitation in part because they understood the resident's medical and functional problems. To be able to send the resident back home was rewarding for staff and reinforced their confidence that the unit delivered high-quality care.

Our preadmission assessment tools have revealed a recent trend toward fewer misdiagnoses. Underdiagnosis of dementia persists, however. Often dementia is ignored, especially in hospitals where primary and secondary diagnosis of dementia can create reimbursement problems (because of diagnosis-related groups [DRGs]). Even the trend to underdiagnosis may be shifting, however, and the reported prevalence of Alzheimer's disease and other dementia diagnoses is climbing.

In 1987 the federal government, under the new Omnibus Budget Reconciliation Act (OBRA), began requiring preadmission screening of nursing home residents for mental illness and mental retardation, in order to eliminate inappropriate placement in nursing homes. This applies to all residents, whether they are discharged from hospitals, are transferred from other nursing institutions, or come directly from home. People with Alzheimer's disease and other progressive dementias are excluded from the extensive screening process. Therefore, it is tempting to alter a diagnosis from mental illness/mental retardation to dementia in order to obtain nursing home placement for a person who is difficult to place. This has resulted in an increased rate of false dementia diagnoses, especially among mentally ill residents who exhibit similar behavior symptoms to dementia residents. Therefore, a nursing home provider should be sure that a prospective dementia unit resident has dementia and not some form of mental illness.

Discharge criteria are also important. Without discharge criteria a unit's resident population becomes progressively less ambulatory until eventually it contains largely residents with end-stage dementia. Thus, programs that aim at serving the higher-functioning, more behaviorally disruptive population must provide a mechanism to decide when a resident no longer represents that subset of dementia residents. Some programs are reluctant to be precise about discharge criteria because they fear that families will avoid placement in a program that is likely to move residents. Others believe that discharge criteria are simply inappropriate. These providers are more likely to keep residents on units throughout the course of the disease under the philosophy that continuity of care will be disrupted if the resident is relocated. In our experience, however, high-quality care can be continued when mechanisms are in place to facilitate a smooth transfer.

Hillhaven chose to implement a very specific set of discharge criteria (table 8-1). These encourage transfer to another area of the facility or discharge from the facility when a resident's condition reaches a defined level.

Adopting complementing admission and discharge criteria encourages homogeneity of the population in the dementia unit, with residents functioning at about the same level. Homogeneity promotes staffing efficiency, because staff are able to develop skills that primarily concentrate on psychosocial, behavioral interventions. Staff skills are not split between the extensive nursing care demands of advanced dementia residents and the more psychosocial demands of higher-functioning residents. A contributing factor to staff work stress ("burnout") may be the feeling of being pulled in too many directions. Maintaining a limited range of resident needs in the dementia unit can greatly reduce this feeling.

Enforcing admission and discharge criteria has direct benefits for the residents. When levels of care are mixed, the more active, ambulatory residents can interfere with care of the resident with more advanced dementia. Attempting to be helpful, for example, a higher functioning resident may untie a more advanced resident's restraint, causing a serious injury. If the facility is structured to deliver services by levels of care needed, as most are, then it makes sense to transfer more advanced dementia residents to the skilled nursing area, where staff expertise shifts along with the physical environment.

It is not unusual for a transfer to be more traumatic for the family than for the resident. A clear discharge policy communicated at the time of admission helps prepare families for the transition when it takes place. After all, no one likes surprises. It is important, however, to keep families involved in the program structure they have become accustomed to. Although a resident has moved off the dementia unit, families should not have to stop interacting with other families and unit staff. If there is a regular support group meeting that a family has been attending, they should continue to attend as long as it benefits them. Remaining sensitive to family support issues is critical; continuity of care should apply to family needs as well as resident needs.

Well-defined admission and discharge criteria also help move inappropriate residents to a more appropriate setting. Sometimes, even with structured admission criteria, residents can be inappropriately placed. Hillhaven occasionally has experienced situations where a resident has a classic, textbook medical evaluation and is diagnosed with dementia and then is later found to have a drug-induced delirium or a treatable depression. In such cases, well-trained staff and medical consultants are able to reassess the resident as function changes. Thus, residents sometimes improve, are reevaluated, and go home.

Second, no matter how good a program is, some residents cannot benefit even though appropriately diagnosed. Unfortunately, an occasional resident may be so combative that he or she cannot be managed, despite staff's best efforts, without constant use of chemical and physical restraints. This is likely to occur in a community where a dementia unit has an excellent reputation for treating severe behavioral problems and frequently receives community referrals of difficult cases.

For example, in some Hillhaven units where staff do an excellent job of managing difficult behaviors, the population of young males with early Alzheimer's disease and aggressive, sometimes violent behavior, has begun to climb. One unit contained three (of 20) residents with a history of dementia pugilistica. These three men were young (early 60s), and all were former boxers. Staff worked diligently to develop behavioral interventions, yet the three men interfered with care so frequently that they infringed on others' right to a safe environment.

It is usually possible for a unit to accommodate one, maybe two residents with extreme behavioral problems. But when a few disruptive residents cause unit staff to disregard functional problems in the others, that unit is headed for trouble. In situations like this, staff must learn that the benefit of the majority of residents depends upon a manageable balance of functional impairments and behavioral problems. Otherwise, a unit may find itself unable to minimize chemical and physical restraints. All admission criteria should include questions that deal with these issues, and the discharge criteria should reinforce the dementia unit's right to treat only those it can care for under the program's mission.

There is obviously never an easy solution to these problems. But without admission and discharge criteria, families and state officials may object to a transfer out of the facility or even to another area of the building, especially if the resident is viewed as difficult to place. As a provider you have ultimate responsibility to prove that you are unable to deliver care based on specific criteria. Without those criteria your arguments for transfer or discharge are significantly weakened.

STAFF TRAINING

After identifying and admitting a resident population appropriate for your program's goals and level of care, you must make sure that staff can deliver the care you promise. Teaching behavioral problem solving is not an easy task. Nursing schools rarely include such skills training in their curriculum. Furthermore, until very recently, state laws have not specified nurse assistant training for the care of dementia residents. The new federal OBRA laws, which require specific nurse assistant training in all states, are the first national attempt to address staff training in nursing homes. Regardless of whether or not a nursing home has a dementia unit, the new laws require nursing homes to address care issues surrounding the disease when training nurse aides.

While the new OBRA law helps address the issue of staff training, it does not spell out exactly what that training should be. Some may argue that this is a drawback, but it could also be considered an asset. Very little information is available about training staff to work with dementia residents. It is dangerous to assume that the type of training makes a difference in how staff care for dementia residents because there has been so little training to begin with. A preliminary evaluation of Hillhaven's dementia unit training program suggests that didactic information on dementia is less important than hands-on training and case examples in substituting behavioral interventions for chemical and physical restraints. Table 8.2 presents a recommended curriculum for training nursing personnel working in dementia units based on Hillhaven's staff training program.

The time and resources needed to adequately train staff are considerable. Added benefits may be lower staff turnover and fewer staff needed to do the job. For these reasons, any dementia unit should invest in a good training program. But facility staff should have the right to set their own training agenda, at least until answers are found about what works and what doesn't work. More research attention needs to be given to evaluating the effectiveness of different training programs for nursing home staff caring for dementia residents.

TABLE 8.2   A Recommended Lesson Plan for Training the Nursing Staff
of a Dementia Unit

Subject	Classroom Instruction	Participatory Instruction
Causes of memory loss	Film (e.g., *Silent Changes in the Brain*) or presentation by medical consultant (15–30 min)	Observe a resident with dementia for 5 min, then discuss as small group (15–30 min)
Medical and psychiatric evaluation	Presentation by medical consultant or case examples from the unit (15–30 min)	Review organization of medical chart; observe administration of Mini-Mental State[a] (15–30 min)
Helping families decide about placement	Film (e.g., *What Shall We Do with Mother?*) or presentation by the person doing admissions (15–30 min)	Role-play a distraught spouse calling for information and coming for an initial visit (15–30 min)
Transfer to the dementia unit	Final preparations for moving; relocation trauma; dealing with families and residents; admission procedures (30–60 min)	Role-play preadmission assessment; observe a preadmission interview; observe an experienced nursing assistant with a new admission (1–2 hr)
Involving the resident's family	Day-to-day strategies; family support groups; handling complaints; legal concerns (60–90 min)	Have nursing assistant attend family support group; role-play a complaining family member; discuss case problems as a group (2–4 hr)
Day-to-day nursing care	Verbal and nonverbal communication; special issues in dressing, bathing, and feeding dementia residents (60–90 min)	Have trainee spend time with experienced nursing assistant; simulate sensory losses with ear plugs and vaseline-smeared glasses; hands-on care working with the nursing educator; discuss problem cases (2–4 hr)
Managing common behavioral problems	Incontinence, sexual acting out, hostility, wandering, rummaging, insomnia, aggressiveness, agitation (60–90 min)	Discuss problem cases in a small group; encourage staff to write up case histories of innovative ways of handling problem behaviors and circulate the winning cases regionally

TABLE 8.2   Continued

Subject	Classroom Instruction	Participatory Instruction
		(Hillhaven's Sherlock Holmes Award program)
Problem-solving when disturbing behaviors arise	General strategies for approaching behavioral problems, including a comprehensive history that searches for causes/precipitating factors (60–90 min)	Role playing and case discussions; team meetings are an excellent setting (2–4 hr)
Nutritional problems and feeding	Metabolic requirements; causes of poor eating; evaluation of the resident with weight loss; organizing the feeding environment to minimize distractions; dealing with agitation, eating inappropriate objects, playing with food, and other problems (30–60 min)	Observe a feeding session and discuss; manage problem feeders with the instructor (1–2 hr)
Activities programming	Presentation by unit activities director; activities as everyone's responsibility (30–60 min)	Planning and leading a program, under supervision of the activities director; discussion of individual interests and skills that could be used (1–2 hr)
Common medications	Presentation by consultant physician or pharmacist; concentrate on tranquilizers, cholinergics, sedative/hypnotics, cardiovascular drugs, and antidepressants (15–30 min)	Review medication lists of one or more new admissions, discussing indications, effects, and possible adverse effects (1–2 hr)
Staff support and enhancement	Sources of job stress; role of management; dealing with staff turnover and job stress (60–90 min)	Discussion of cases and personal concerns in facilitated small groups (1–2 hr)

(*continued*)

TABLE 8.2 Continued

Subject	Classroom Instruction	Participatory Instruction
Care of the end-stage patient; why residents are moved off the unit	Letting go of residents who must leave the unit; changing care requirements (15–30 min)	Visiting advanced care patients in other parts of the facility; observing advanced care; discussion of feelings when a resident leaves

Source: Adapted from Orr, N., and Reifler, B. B. 1985. *Alzheimer's Disease in the Nursing Home: A Staff Training Manual.* Tacoma, Wash.: Hillhaven Corporation.
[a]Folstein, M. F., Folstein, S., and McHugh, P. R. 1975. Mini-Mental state: Practical method for grading cognitive state of patients for the clinician. *Journal of Psychiatric Research* 12:189–98.

MEDICAL LEADERSHIP

Hillhaven facilities hire a medical consultant for every dementia unit above and beyond the medical director for the facility. This physician rarely has attending responsibilities for residents and is actually discouraged from assuming any. The primary function of this consultant is to advise staff and family and to assist other physicians. The medical consultant is responsible for assuring the accuracy of dementia diagnoses and directly advising staff about care policies. Consultants who perform their role properly are welcomed by attending physicians because they often minimize overuse or inappropriate use of their time. The critical issue is to hire someone in this position who supports the unit's philosophy of care and will devote four or five hours a month to help make it work.

SOCIAL ACTIVITIES ON THE UNIT

Now that the resident population has been determined, the staff trained in new behavioral techniques, and medical leadership secured, you must develop the programs necessary to deliver optimal care. A body of knowledge is accumulating about the design and implementation of successful activities programs for dementia units. The details are presented in chapters 12 and 13.

The activities on a specialized unit need to do more than provide a social outlet. These programs should function as an internal day care program. They must be a focal point for preventing behavioral problems and encouraging resident self-esteem. Without the right activity programming behavioral management in lieu of chemical and physical restraints is nearly impossible.

For residents with problem behaviors, staff must design a management plan that addresses motives. Through an understanding of a person's past and the development of an appropriate outlet or activity, behavioral problems can often be avoided. For example, we had a resident on a dementia unit who tried to leave the unit every day at sunset. She would cry and eventually become so upset that she would strike out at other residents and staff who tried to distract her or hinder her leaving. Telling her she need not worry about home now that she lived at the facility only upset her more. In the past, she had raised five children and had never once in 30 years missed preparing meals. Once staff understood this, they were able to work out an appropriate activity to prevent her agitation from escalating. Every afternoon the activity director or a nursing assistant sat with her and reviewed family photo albums, discussing her career as a mother and housewife until it was time for dinner. The problem behavior quickly subsided.

This example illustrates the importance activity programming can play in making life meaningful for dementia residents and in controlling behavioral problems associated with the disease. In the best programs the division between nursing and activity staff becomes blurred. Activity staff often get involved in the traditional nursing domain, such as hygiene and grooming. Similarly, nursing staff on a unit should not hesitate to lead an activity, especially if they have particular skills they enjoy sharing. Successful activity programming involves nursing and activities working together to build resident self-esteem, to prevent behavioral problems, and to manage problems effectively when they occur.

This focus on activities takes a considerable amount of time and effort. It usually should be the primary responsibility of a single person. Often, a full-time person is necessary. Assisted by other staff and volunteers, this person can provide activities throughout the residents' waking hours. The activity staff should make sure that nursing staff are comfortable conducting activities without supervision when no activity staff is present. Administration should allocate the time necessary for nursing staff to fill in whenever necessary and to participate on a regular basis.

To share caregiving responsibilities does not come naturally and requires an organized effort on everyone's part. One way of addressing this issue is to include it in the staff training program. The message should then be reinforced with specific assignments in nursing, such as an activity a week for all nursing staff. It can be a fun way of learning the psychosocial aspects of caregiving.

OPERATIONAL COSTS

Day-to-day operational costs must be anticipated and managed. As discussed earlier in this chapter, initial construction costs should always be calculated before deciding to start a dementia unit because they weigh heavily on the feasibility of the overall program. The greatest costs are for labor, however, especially as the program's census is building.

There are no magic ladders or ratios that say how many staff are needed to care for dementia residents. Much depends on the population of residents you decide to serve. Like a generic activities program, a generic staffing formula does not exist. A provider must be flexible and must understand that the program may need adjustment as it grows. Operating within a staffing range often makes the best sense. Hillhaven staffs its dementia units within a range of minimal to maximal direct nursing hours given to residents. This is called nursing hours per resident day (NHPRD). It does not include administrative time or other department time, such as activities. The Hillhaven dementia unit range, 2.6–3.0 NHPRD, is the same or higher than required skilled nursing care levels set by states. We established this policy because we believed that to accomplish our mission of no chemical or physical restraints we had to staff at the skilled care level. This decision was made despite the fact that most Medicaid reimbursement systems view the level of resident care in our units as intermediate or below. It is important, therefore, that whatever staffing ratios you choose, you can account for the reimbursement differences within the state system, usually with private pay revenues.

The second major labor expense is in activities because caring for demented residents requires a psychosocial focus. Activity staff costs are proportional to experience and relevant degrees. Most facilities would like to hire occupational therapists, music therapists, or other appropriate degreed professionals but are limited in their ability to do so either because they cannot afford to pass the cost to the consumer or because a professional with interest and expertise is not available.

The third major labor cost comes from the medical consultant you hire. This is a cost not reimbursed by Medicare or Medicaid. Unless you use your consultant extensively, however, the per day cost to your residents is minimal and well worth the investment.

Often facilities express concern about increased labor costs in the areas of housekeeping, dietary services, laundry, and maintenance. Our programs do not experience greater cost in these areas than is experienced in the general facility. However, they might if Hillhaven operated buildings entirely for the care of dementia residents. As it is, these labor needs are not significant enough to warrant distinct, higher levels of staffing.

In addition to labor, the cost of dietary services appears to be higher in our dementia units. The vast majority of these increased costs pay for supplementary snacks between meals. Because our residents are more active than the average nursing home resident (in some cases, they are hyperactive), they need more calories. In addition, many activity programs use food. For example, a unit may have a cooking class three times a week for the former housewives who can still benefit therapeutically from participating in making goodies for other residents. Finally, it is probably wise to maintain a pantry on the unit for staff and families so that snacks can be available as needed. A pantry helps to keep labor costs in dietary services down.

Marketing costs are likely to be greatest in the first year of unit operation. Failing to plan for them can create financial problems. The development of brochures and written materials, advertisement of the new services, and staff recruitment can add up quickly. Such expenses can wreak havoc in a budget for months after opening the unit. Plan carefully and, if necessary, with the help of outside professionals.

Once all major costs of day-to-day operations have been budgeted, the size of the dementia unit becomes critical. Often the physical plant limits the number of beds that can be accommodated. There is some opinion that units should be kept small—approximately 12 beds or less (Gwyther and Mace 1989). While this may be ideal, from a cost standpoint it is usually impractical. The fewer the beds, the greater the cost to the consumer. In some cases the costs of operating a special unit can be passed on equally to all residents whether they use the special unit or not, but often this is not the case. Usually, dementia unit costs are shared only by those who actually use the service. As in any market, a seller of service has to be sure the service is competitive and affordable. Furthermore, no operator, whether for profit or not for profit, can afford to lose large sums of money.

Based in part on cost considerations, Hillhaven tends to operate dementia units that contain around 25 beds. This number provides an effective compromise between efficient staffing and a therapeutic environment. It is neither too large nor too small. Larger units are less expensive but usually become difficult to manage because the residents react negatively to crowds and noise. Hillhaven's experience is that residents in large, crowded situations become behaviorally difficult to manage, thus defeating the program's mission.

Setting goals for census development is important. If you are starting with a new unit that is completely empty on the starting date, expect it to take approximately eight months to reach full capacity. Much of census development depends on what type of mix you hope to attract and what type of marketing plan you have in effect. Hillhaven's experience indicates that the first few months are slow and that the pace picks up after the fourth month.

To avoid inappropriate admissions, specific admission criteria should be adhered to. How rapidly a new unit fills depends in part on how strictly these criteria are followed, but developing a population slowly pays lasting benefits. If residents are carefully selected, turnover is minimal. Alzheimer's residents in need of primarily psychosocial care and other dementia residents tend to live longer than other nursing home residents. Good caregiving with few chemical and physical restraints not only provides quality care but probably increases residents' life span.

Administrative Structure

INTEGRATION WITH OTHER AREAS OF THE FACILITY

A dementia unit in a nursing facility in many ways functions as a small, independent entity, separate from the rest of the facility. It is a separate area distinctly marked off from the rest of the building by secured doors. There are a separate nursing station and separate dining and activity spaces. The residents and staff rarely leave the unit except for special facility events or scheduled outings. As a result, it is easy for a unit to develop its own unique, cohesive, and caring work environment. The greatest benefit of such an atmosphere, when it functions well, is that staff turnover is lowered. The biggest drawback is that it can create jealousies and strained working relationships elsewhere in the facility.

This is a fine line to walk. One one hand you will want to instill the mission of the program so that staff, residents, and families work together cohesively. People associated with the unit absolutely need to feel special. But feeling special is different than being perceived as "better." This is where the administrative structure of a unit becomes critical.

Staff on the unit must be organized so that job responsibilities overlap or are shared with staff outside the unit. For example, a unit coordinator may be responsible for training staff but may share the responsibility of staffing the unit with the facility's nursing director. An example that has been controversial for our programs, is whether the activity coordinator on the dementia unit should be supervised by the facility activity department head or by the unit coordinator. We recommend that the activity director for the building have direct supervision responsibility in order to ensure that department head's continued involvement. An informal line of authority exists between the nurse coordinator and the activities coordinator, but each remain responsible directly to a department head. This structure ensures the direct involvement of people with responsibilities outside the dementia unit. It also maintains the discipline-specific responsibility required by state and federal governments.

In some situations the unit coordinator may be directly supervised by the facility administrator instead of by his or her department head. This is particularly appropriate if the coordinator has a variety of responsibilities, including direct care, marketing, and public speaking on behalf of the facility. Still, coordinators should never be without a relationship to their primary discipline.

You may decide to make the unit coordinator a department head in order to establish the authority of that position and to keep the coordinator actively involved in decision making throughout the building. However, in most cases this should not be necessary. After all, how many department heads can there be? If the coordinator of a dementia unit is given such status, the head nurse of the rehabilitation unit may well ask for it. These types of conflict can be avoided by maintaining clear and distinct communications within disciplines.

THE UNIT COORDINATOR

Who the coordinator should be is another decision that can have a powerful influence in your program. A dementia unit director should have clear leadership responsibilities and feel ownership for the success of the program. Hillhaven has a wide variety of programs led by people with diverse backgrounds (e.g., activities, nursing, and social work). Flexibility in this area is important, and decisions should depend on the personnel resources of a facility.

Major problems can arise if the unit coordinator's position is not handled according to basic personnel management principles. For example, assigning someone without a clear job description or adding the job to other responsibilities can doom the position from the beginning. A coordinator who is poorly supervised and managed ultimately leads to a poorly operated unit.

In the start-up phase it is important to decide what kind of leadership your program needs, how best to orchestrate it, and then to hire someone early on. For example, your area may have a good deal of competition and a significant number of empty nursing home beds. You may be beginning your unit as an entirely new program without transferring residents from inside your facility to the unit. You may have also figured that the cost of the program will require a significant private pay mix to cover your costs. Such a situation demands that your coordinator have time to work outside the facility, unless you have someone else in house with the time and skills necessary to do marketing and public education.

THE ACTIVITIES STAFF

The second most important personnel decision is selection of the activities staff. In a start-up situation, you may decide to build activity hours based on your population of residents. This is not only cost efficient but assures that nursing staff learn from the beginning to share responsibility with the activities department.

Start-up for an activities program is often quite expensive because of staffing costs. However, it is well worth the investment to absorb the costs up front for the benefits when your program is at full occupancy. A new program is difficult because of the need for residents to adjust to a new environment. Most take weeks to two months to begin making the transition. It is a time when resident care can be quite difficult and staffing is critical. Unless staffing is adequate you are likely to begin experiencing staff turnover and possibly an increase in worker compensation claims. A new program can ill afford to start off on the wrong foot with the loss of key personnel. No amount of outside marketing will change the problems you create for yourself by staffing inadequately.

Marketing and Public Relations

I have attempted to stress throughout this chapter the importance of doing the program "right" and for the primary purpose of providing quality care. There are no gimmicks that will magically help your facility's census or its percentage of private pay residents. Families who can afford good care are extremely particular and, as a rule, quite well educated about nursing care services.

As consumer education improves for Alzheimer's families and as more nursing homes offer specialized services, the pressures to deliver high-quality service also increase. A good, strategically placed advertisement may get families in the door, but they won't buy an inferior product. Marketing and public relations run beyond good advertisements and fancy open houses and, in the end, boil down to high quality and commitment.

REACHING POTENTIAL NEW RESIDENTS

Hillhaven's experience is that families and community support services are naturally skeptical of intentions to develop and operate a dementia unit. The best response is to handle this view as a challenge. Be prepared to prove your intentions. By all means be honest with everyone you work with about what you are going to do. Then follow through. Do not promise what you cannot deliver, and you will receive realistic support in return. This sounds simplistic. It is easy, however, to find yourself in a situation where families and referral services begin telling you what to do and how to do it, especially when you are trying to meet peoples' needs. To avoid such situations you should begin your marketing efforts with education.

Families and potential referrals want to know what your program is intended to do. Their primary concern is clinical care; so you must be able to use terminology that they understand. Brochures and literature should not only speak to your mission but also to how you expect to accomplish it. Avoid jargon and generalizations; be prepared to explain whatever you have written.

You will want to target marketing efforts to specific services and people whom you consider likely referral sources. Traditionally, nursing homes have received the majority of their admissions from hospitals. Hospitals are an unlikely referral source for a new dementia unit, however, unless that unit is interested in treating advanced Alzheimer's residents with multiple disabilities.

Most potential dementia unit admissions live at home. In fact, 79 percent of Hillhaven's special care unit admissions come directly from home. Before admission, they were usually cared for by their spouse or one of their children, although a surprising number were living alone.

Identifying these potential residents is not easy but is nevertheless important. Sometimes hospitals see these people because of a crisis, but a large number are identified through nonmedical community services such as police, fire departments, or public transportation systems. Thus, providing education about your services to these groups may prove beneficial. Seek out opportunities to meet with staff of nonmedical community services that can identify at-risk people.

GAINING COMMUNITY SUPPORT

Many nursing homes start by marketing to their local Alzheimer's Association. This is a likely source of referral, but only if you approach the organization properly and with respect for its position in the community. Showing up just to attend a support group meeting means little to an organization that is often short on volunteers and struggling to meet all the needs of families. As a former president of an Alzheimer's Association chapter, I can assure you that staff never looked favorably on nursing home providers and other service organizations who just passed out business cards or brochures and told us how wonderful their services were. We expected everyone who wanted help from us to be willing to join us in the fight against this dreaded disease. The message here is quite simple: be prepared to give of yourself and your expertise. This does not necessarily mean money. Discover the organization's needs and try to do what you can to meet them. Eventually you will begin to receive the support you need.

An example involves the complicated issue of health care reimbursement. One of the greatest gifts you can give members of the Alzheimer's Association may be education. Most families do not understand their Medicaid, Medicare, or private payment systems and under what conditions their relative might be eligible for certain programs. Furthermore, families are not well educated about the regulations that govern the nursing home industry or how reimbursement systems affect the provider. Few facilities work with families to understand. Yet a basic principle of marketing is to help others to understand what you do, why you do it, what you can do for them, and how they can best work with you.

Facilities often make the mistake of using a lot of media advertising to market a service, especially if the competition is doing so. This can be an expensive avenue that should be pursued carefully. If you advertise, make sure that your staff is prepared to answer inquiries and to follow up on them. Often money is wasted when a successful radio blitz generates inquiries that never materialize into admissions because phone calls are not handled properly.

Getting the word out is not the same as converting inquiries into admissions. Marketing often focuses energy on what is outside your building. However, it is what is inside your building and how you present yourself that will convert an inquiry into an admission. Knowing how to give a family a tour is very important; all staff must convey the same important message.

If your program is a novelty in your community, you will probably get inquiries from people who are unlikely to have an impact on your admissions. As a rule we allow few people other than families of dementia patients to tour our units. Dementia unit tours must respect residents' rights and allow staff to maintain an organized caring environment.

Support has to be earned; it cannot be bought. Recently, I received a call from a Hillhaven facility asking the company to make a relatively large donation to the local Alzheimer's Association. When I inquired about the facility's working relationship with the association to date, the administrator informed me that it was poor. No family inquiries had been received from the association; no one from the organization had attended our open house; and the local association newsletter had written a negative report on specialized nursing home units. The facility believed that by giving the association financial support it would turn its opinion around. I denied the request for funds until the facility administrator met with the association's director to discuss the poor working relationship and came to an agreement on how to improve it. Ultimately, issues were resolved and improvements made to the point that many inquiries now come from the association and our dementia unit coordinator is on the association's board of directors. The point to be made is that no amount of money is going to resolve bad working relations.

WHEN A NEW UNIT OPENS

A variety of things can be done to officially announce your new dementia unit. Many facilities like to send announcements and have an official open house. The most successful facilities will have already had several reasons for contacting those people receiving announcements or invitations.

People come to open houses for two reasons: curiosity or support. By far the preferred reason is support. When people have been involved in what you are doing they are more likely to send referrals and work to see you succeed. The commitment is greater because they are involved. You must work with the community throughout dementia unit development in order for your open house to succeed. An open house is a marvelous time to recognize the efforts of all involved and to reemphasize your commitment to helping victims of this disease and their families.

Once you begin admitting residents, it is tempting to fill a new unit quickly. Do not, however, allow admissions to exceed your staffing levels and staff training. Stagger admissions and pay attention to your coordinator's concerns. Relocation is quite traumatic for residents with Alzheimer's, and the behavioral problems are always greater immediately after placement than after a few weeks of residency. Prepare families, residents, and staff as much as possible before an admission, and avoid more than two admissions a day or five a week. If you have done a super job of marketing your program, evaluating prospective residents as much as several months before opening, this should not be much of a problem. Most dementia units fill slowly because referral services and families are skeptical. Do not be surprised if it takes four to six months to fill a 25-bed unit. If you do it properly, taking your time and prescreening admissions, you will lessen the stress and strain on everyone.

Marketing services beyond the open house is critical but is often overlooked when the responsibilities of care start picking up. Have a measurable plan for ongoing contact, and consider marketing as every employee's concern. Keep files on contacts. Pay particular attention to people who did not come to the open house. When you get a referral, follow up with a thank you. Some programs get family permission to use a resident's name and a short "progress note" about his or her adjustment to the new home. This type of follow-up is especially good to provide to physicians, who too frequently get negative feedback or no feedback at all. Whatever inroads you can make with physicians to help them better understand what you are doing is worth the investment because families often turn to physicians as the primary source of help.

MAINTAINING GOOD RELATIONSHIPS WITH FAMILIES

Sometimes facilities think that in order to project the right market image they must have a support group for families. Support groups are not for everyone and are not easily established or run. A support group does not necessarily help your market image, especially if the service is already offered in your community. In fact, duplicating a service may harm your residents with other service providers in the community who may view themselves as experts in their areas. Your objectives should be to find out what your families and community want, to complement other services, and to fill gaps in the continuum of care.

Maintaining good relationships with families is vital. Inevitably some families will not be happy with your services. Some complaints will be justified and others will not. All complaints should be considered equally important, however. For example, a family member was quite verbal about what a bad job she thought one of our dementia units was doing. She was not interested in moving her relative, even though we offered to help when we could not meet all her demands. She spoke out at local support groups and complained to anyone who would listen. We thought her complaints were exaggerated and assumed that others would as well until our census began to drop. It took a tremendous effort to undo the damage, however unjustified, with supporters who took the woman's comments at face value. The facility learned that complaints, no matter how absurd, need to be resolved.

No matter how much families and the community appreciate your service, state survey teams responsible for licensure and certification may not receive it well. If you want to contest survey results, the support you receive from others in the community may make a difference. It is wise to consider involving state officials in the planning and implementation of your unit. That way you are in a better position to communicate your intent and clarify your clinical approach to care. The time to gain support for your program is in the planning stage, not during the survey process.

In summary, involving your staff in all areas of marketing and public relations can be fun and a rewarding experience. All of us, regardless of our line of work, welcome the opportunity to share what we do and what we know in a positive setting. Use all your staff in your efforts, whether they work directly with residents on the unit or not. Everyone has the right to be proud of the part played in delivering care to Alzheimer's residents and their families and should be given the opportunity to share their pride with others.

References

Gwyther, L., and Mace, N. 1989. *Selecting a Nursing Home with a Dedicated Dementia Unit*. Chicago: Alzheimer's Association.
Jackson, M. E., Drugovich, M. L., Fretwell, M. D., Spector, W. D., Sternberg, J., and Rosenstein, R. B. 1989. Prevalence and correlates of disruptive behavior in the nursing home. *Journal of Aging and Health* 1: 349–69.
Panella, J. J. 1987. *Day Care Programs for Alzheimer's Disease and Related Disorders*. New York: Demo Publications.

Sheridan, C. 1987. *Failure-free Activities for the Alzheimer's Unit.* Oakland, Calif.: Cottage Books.

Yankelovich, Skelley, and White/Clancy, Shulman, Inc. 1986. *Caregivers of Patients with Dementia.* Contract report prepared for the Office of Technology Assessment, United States Congress. Washington, D.C.: U.S. Government Printing Office.

9

Common Problems in Developing, Implementing, and Maintaining a Dementia Unit

LAURA J. MATHEW AND PHILIP D. SLOANE

Because the concept of a dementia unit is still relatively new for the nursing home industry, we asked administrators of homes with dementia units to review and evaluate their experience. More specifically, we asked administrators (or someone they designated, such as the unit director) for their opinions on why they began such a unit, the greatest benefits and drawbacks of the unit, what they regarded as the ideal unit, what rewards were given to the staff, and what strategies were used for marketing purposes. Their answers were provided to us in the form of narrative responses. Although the responses were based on personal experience, we found many similarities among them and believed that this information may be helpful to those considering a new unit. This chapter summarizes our findings.

Why Dementia Units Are Begun

Administrative staff commonly described an unmet need that required action. With a large percentage of their residents suffering from dementia, it had become clear that special programming was necessary. Demented residents required a different approach, they believed. Those who were cognitively intact often complained about the behavior of demented residents; their wandering, rummaging, and frequent need for direction were bothersome.

In the words of one administrator, the unit was started "to help establish a routine for those who could not deal with what appears to them to be mass confusion, but in reality was just normal routine . . . to provide a section for restructuring to the resident's need, not ours."

Some administrators believed that neither the cognitively intact nor the demented could receive humane treatment before the unit was established. Persons who were aware of their surroundings and able to maneuver well complained often of feeling that they were in a psychiatric ward, unable to predict what the day would bring. Demented residents, on the other hand, were usually left behind when activities began and were tied down for a variety of reasons. They seemed to require additional attention from the staff, although little improvement was ever noticed or expected to occur.

Many staff members working in the home also became weary with the situation, although some always seemed to work well with the demented population. These few workers often succeeded where others would not even try. They became the "chosen few" that nursing directors carefully selected and trained for the new dementia unit.

The Greatest Benefits of a Dementia Unit

Relief for families and a more comfortable existence for the demented resident were common benefits attributed to dementia units. Units were sometimes started because no one else would care for the demented in a community. Families were described as being "at the edge of their tolerance."

The plight of family caregivers has been well documented in the literature, through government reports, and the media. Their accounts are familiar to professionals yet somewhat difficult to understand at an emotional level unless the professional has also experienced the day-to-day burden of caring for a demented relative.

Coupled with feelings of desperation are concerns for the well-being of the victim. Families and staff of the home expressed satisfaction at being able to manage a resident with minimal physical or chemical restraints. Without such a specially designed and programmed unit, this more dignified existence may not be possible. The unit provided an area for safe wandering, freedom of expression, acceptance, and flexibility of routines. Emphasis could now be placed on remaining abilities, attempting to improve the overall quality of the victim's life. Common responses are reflected by the following statement of one administrator: "Care is

better supervised, . . . agitation is reduced, . . . abilities are maximized,
. . . families are supported, . . . and our residents receive a quality of life
they would otherwise not experience in most facilities."

The Greatest Drawbacks

A feeling of being different, isolated, or special arose as concerns of
administrative staff. There was a need to balance the unique value of a
special unit against the possibility of isolation from what is more commonly expected and known to occur in a nursing home. Staff, families,
and visitors reacted to the closed doors, the different routines followed,
and the environmental changes. Also, administrative staff described feelings of uncertainty about how to begin and operate a successful unit.
They often welcomed the opportunity to speak with others in this pioneering field.

A few concerns were frequently repeated and are worthy of further
discussion. One such concern is the difficulty of deciding when a resident
is ready to be moved off the unit. Most administrators could define the
criteria for admission of a resident, but discharging was a more difficult
process. Staff members and families had adjusted to the placement of the
resident, and problems arose when this connection was severed.

Another concern involved the great need to provide support for staff
and family members. These persons were stressed; they often responded
by expressing despair and low expectations. There was a constant reminder to address this issue.

A third concern was financial. These units are expensive to operate.
All had to rely in part on private funding because Medicare and Medicaid
have strict limitations on reimbursement to nursing homes. Start-up
costs were high, because new units entailed more space, structural modifications, higher staffing ratios, training of staff, and the development of
procedures for which there were few standards. While some are sus-
pected of marketing their services only to the wealthy, dementia unit
administrators commonly agreed that a good unit is costly and needs
appropriate reimbursement from both private and public sources.

Last, a common concern was the nursing shortage faced by health
facilities everywhere. Nursing homes are constantly competing with other settings to fill vacant positions. Staff turnover was felt to affect adverse-
ly continuity of care, orientation and training costs, and relationships
with family members. While we noted less turnover on the dementia
units than on the comparison units (see chapter 6), the perception that
turnover was problematic seemed to remain among dementia unit administrators.

Still, the administrative staff seemed to persevere. One person acknowledged that "there is a lot of stress, but the love is always over-powering."

Elements of an Ideal Unit

The administrators' concept of an ideal unit seemed to be one that addressed the problems listed above. It included such attributes as more space (especially access to the outdoors), more staff trained in specialties such as social work and recreation therapy assigned exclusively to the dementia unit, and a larger budget to allow for expanded programming.

A unit that could accommodate the varying stages of dementia was a frequent idea. It would also address the problem of discharging a resident into a traditional setting.

The words of one administrator summed up the ideal unit. It would be one "in which the resident is protected from harming himself, but where he may be encouraged to use every skill remaining to live as full a life as possible."

Rewards Given to Staff

Most people we spoke with attached value to staff retention. We were repeatedly told that resources spent on the unit staff were well spent. Rewards for the staff included special recognition through certificates, receptions, and nominations for various achievements and bonuses. One facility devised a system of class reunions after educational programs. Acknowledgment from families was a particularly important reward.

Perhaps the most important reward was a sense of accomplishment. This came in a variety of forms, such as positive reinforcement from superiors, recognition of valuable suggestions made for improving care, and involvement in care planning and unit management. Some homes stated that staff took pride in knowing that their residents received proper care. Others identified the opportunity to learn and be challenged. One person stated that "working with these residents is a reward in itself; . . . many staff members volunteer to work on the unit."

Marketing Strategies

Administrators mentioned a variety of marketing strategies. Some homes stated that absolutely nothing was done. For some of them, the local need was so great that a long waiting list accumulated. Others relied on a good reputation for a steady source of referrals.

However, most facilities had a program for attracting potential residents. This involved publicity in newspapers (in the form of ads or articles written on the subject); participation in television and radio talk shows; taking part in community events, such as setting up a booth at a health fair; and providing community outreach programs. The latter included an Alzheimer's disease speakers' bureau, monthly support group meetings for family members, a journal club open to the community, and tours of the facility conducted by staff.

Brochures were developed by the staff at many homes. These were distributed to hospitals, clinics, government agencies such as area agencies on aging, or local senior citizen groups. Professional organizations, such as the Alzheimer's Association, also received these announcements. When units began operating, professionals were invited to tour the facility at a formal reception or open house.

Another approach included a display of art work created by the residents. Ceramics or quilts made by the more cognitively intact residents of the home were displayed in the community. While these crafts were not made by demented residents, they brought recognition to the home as a whole.

Thus, most of the homes marketed their services. Staff at all levels were encouraged to participate in speaking engagements and to be visible, representing the dementia unit in the community.

The Innovation Continues

The novelty of dementia units is beginning to fade now, and the elements of specialized care are being redefined as services that should be available to all residents in long-term care. Those who pioneered this field, however, began a movement of change and innovation for the industry. Questions remain unanswered, administrators continue to struggle in defining policies, and there is still disagreement among those providing care.

From the administrators' statements, however, one conclusion seems eminent. This movement toward specialized care is firmly embedded in the nursing home industry. The unique benefits and the potential for enhancing the quality of lives far outweigh the problems that are likely to arise. The challenge for caregivers is to provide an environment where the demented person can continue to flourish, given the constraints of the disease.

IV

The Physical Environment

10

Environmental Characteristics of Existing Dementia Units

LAURA J. MATHEW AND PHILIP D. SLOANE

Environments created specifically for the elderly have received more consideration in recent years (Koncelik 1979; Moos and Lemke 1984; Koff 1988). The literature often mentions the need to design an environment that reflects an understanding of the aging process. More specifically, items such as lighting, coloring, noise, and orientation or wayfinding are often brought up as important elements of the surroundings.

These issues are of particular significance when designing a residential space for demented elderly (Calkins 1988; Cohen et al. 1988). Processing sensory input may be difficult for those with cognitive impairment. In combination with loud noise, glare, and obstacles along a pathway, for example, this weakness may cause frustration in a resident. Added stress and behavioral problems may result.

Though little data-based research exists on the impact of the physical environment on the dementing process, there is general consensus that environment plays a role in creating an overall atmosphere conducive to good care (Coons 1985; Hiatt 1979; U.S. Congress 1987.) Thus, we were interested in describing how the environments of dementia units we visited differed from settings providing traditional care.

This chapter discusses findings from our study of 31 dementia units in five states. Study methods are presented in the introduction and Appendix of this volume. The chapter begins with data collected on all nursing homes we visited. A discussion of characteristics of only those facilities that house a dementia unit follows. The chapter ends by comparing the environmental characteristics of the dementia units and comparison units. In particular, it reports our impressions of how therapeutic the environments seemed during our site visits.

Physical Structure of All Facilities Visited

Administrators of the facilities we visited were asked to complete a questionnaire that included items describing the physical structure of nursing homes. Structural components included the following: total area in square feet for residents on the unit, number and type of rooms, bed capacity in the various types of rooms, existence of a separate dining room, existence of a separate activities room, and accessibility to the outdoors. These findings are summarized in tables 10.1, 10.2, and 10.3.

The total area used by residents on the units differed greatly between settings. Dementia units had a mean of 10,851.6 square feet; the comparison units were about twice that size, with a mean of 19,412.6 square feet. However, a total of 965 residents (with a mean census of 35.9) were on the dementia units we visited, compared with 1,883 residents (with a mean census of 59.1) in the comparison units. The actual space per resident was 302.3 square feet for the dementia units, very similar to that for the comparison units, which was 328.5 square feet. The smaller size of the dementia units, however, allowed for more control over factors such as noise level and the tendency of cognitively impaired residents to become more confused when placed in large units.

With regard to the total number of rooms on the units, distinct differences were found between the two settings. Dementia units had a mean of 21.3 rooms, and comparison units, 34.2 rooms. This difference is explained again by a larger resident census on comparison units, which obviously required more rooms. Dementia units tended to have fewer rooms overall, indicating that their intention may have been to limit the number of residents.

There were few differences in the actual number of private rooms available. The mean number of private rooms on the dementia units was 7.8, with a range of 0 to 32. On the comparison units, the mean was identical (7.8), although the range was wider, from 0 to 94 private rooms available. The wider range of private rooms on the comparison units also resulted in part from the larger capacity of these units.

However, a more substantial proportion of the bed capacity on the dementia units was made available in the form of private rooms (see table

TABLE 10.1   Structural Characteristics of Units

	Dementia Units (N = 26)	Comparison Units (N = 24)
Square footage		
Mean	10,851.6	19,412.6
Range	2044–40,000	2000–58,000
Total no. of rooms		
Mean	21.3	34.2
Range	6–57	4–95
Number of private rooms		
Mean	7.8	7.8
Range	0–32	0.94

TABLE 10.2   Bed Capacity in Private and Nonprivate Rooms

	No. (%) of Dementia Units	No. (%) of Comparison Units	p
Nonprivate rooms	844 (78.4)	1639 (86.7)	<.001
Private rooms	232 (21.6)	250 (13.2)	

TABLE 10.3   Units with Separate Dining and Activities Rooms and Access to Outdoors (%)

	Dementia Units (N = 30)	Comparison Units (N = 32)	p
Separate dining room			
Yes	90%	66%	<.05
No	10	34	
Separate activities room			
Yes	86.7	71	.13
No	13.3	29	
Access to outdoors			
Yes	86.7	84.4	.80
No	13.3	15.6	

10.2). Dementia units had approximately 21.6 percent of their total bed capacity in private rooms; comparison units had 13.2 percent. The difference was statistically significant ($p < .001$). Conversations with staff indicated that this emphasis on private rooms made certain resident conditions, such as rummaging, pillaging, or hoarding, more manageable.

A separate dining room for the residents on a unit adds greatly to the ease with which residents can be escorted to meals. The dementia units more often had separate dining rooms; 90 percent answered in the affirmative. About 66 percent of the comparison units employed this feature in their design. The difference was statistically significant ($p < .05$). Table 10.3 lists our findings in terms of the percentage of units having a separate dining room, activities room, and courtyard.

Likewise, a separate activities area may increase the possibility of greater involvement of the residents. While a larger percentage of dementia units answered in the affirmative (86.7 percent versus 71 percent), this difference was not significant ($p = .134$). It may be that a separate activities area has gained more acceptance than a separate dining room. More nursing homes overall are now including separate activities space for the residents of a particular unit. Consequently no major differences are being seen among facilities.

Administrators who reported having a separate area for activities in the unit were also asked to specify the number of square feet in that area. We found major differences between settings. Dementia units had a mean area of 1,337.5 square feet for their activity rooms; the range was 192 to 12,000 square feet. In contrast, the comparison units had a mean of 457.4 square feet for their activity rooms; the range here was from 0 to 1,944 square feet. Dementia units tended to have about twice the space set aside for activities areas. Because their average census was smaller, this meant that dementia units offered far more space per resident for activities. Lastly, all facilities were asked about the existence of a courtyard, solarium, or other protected area that made the outdoors accessible to unit residents. No differences were seen in the responses, with 86.7 percent of the dementia units and 84.4 percent of the comparison units reporting such areas. When asked if residents had to be accompanied by staff to use outdoor areas, 50 percent of the dementia units answered in the affirmative. About 53.6 percent of the comparison unit administrators replied similarly. Thus, the reported existence of an outdoor area did not differ between settings, and actual usage may also not differ because of other factors such as the need for staff accompaniment.

However, we will show later in this chapter that our site visits did not confirm the reported accessibility of outdoor areas. Direct accessibility of outdoor areas was more frequent among dementia units. This finding

TABLE 10.4   Characteristics of Facilities with Dementia Units ($N = 30$)

Age of building (yr)	
Mean	15.3
Median	15.0
Range	1–40
Age of dementia unit (yr)	
Mean	4.6
Median	2.29
Range	0.58–25.3
No. of facilities with more than one unit	3

Note: This information is based on data from 30 units; one dementia unit did not complete the questionnaire.

illustrates the drawbacks of questionnaire data and the importance of direct observation.

Structural Qualities Specific to Dementia Units

Administrators of the dementia units in our sample were asked a set of additional questions regarding their facilities. These included the age of the building, the date the dementia unit actually got established, and whether more than one unit was designated for dementia residents. Also, we asked whether the unit was built specifically as a dementia unit, and if not, whether it had been renovated. Lastly, we asked if the dementia unit was physically isolated from the rest of the facility. Tables 10.4 and 10.5 display our findings.

There was diversity in the ages of the buildings and the programs administered. The mean age of the buildings housing our sample of dementia units was 15.3 years. The newest building was only 1 year old; the oldest was 40 years old. Likewise, the age of the dementia units varied greatly, the newest having been established only seven months before our visit and the oldest unit being more than 25 years old. However, the mean age of the dementia units was 4.6 years and the median was 2.29 years, indicating that, for the most part, the units we chose were still fairly new.

Only three facilities (out of 31) had more than one dementia unit. However, through our informal conversations with administrative staff, we learned that several were considering establishing other units. Reasons cited included long waiting lists and difficulty in transferring re-

TABLE 10.5   Structural Features of the Dementia Units ($N = 29$)

	No. (%) of Units
Specifically built as dementia unit	6 (21)
Renovated before unit established	17 (59)
Converted without renovation	6 (21)
Physically isolated from rest of facility	25 (87)
Not physically isolated	4 (13)

Note: For two units, data on these physical features were incomplete or absent.

sidents who could benefit more from another type of dementia unit.

Six out of 29 dementia units (21 percent) had been built specifically as specialized areas. These units had incorporated several design features that are often associated with dementia units. For example, they were likely to contain well-defined spaces designated for dining, activities, or small group interactions. Of the 23 units that had not been built specifically for dementia programs, most (73.9 percent) had undergone renovation.

Last, when asked whether the dementia unit was isolated, the vast majority, or 86.7 percent, replied in the affirmative. Isolation was usually achieved through such devices as closed (but unlocked) doors, a variety of alarm systems, dutch doors, or some type of divider placed across a hallway. A few units relied on alarm systems placed on the ankles of the residents themselves, eliminating the need for physical isolation of the unit through closed doors. However, most staff we spoke with alluded to the benefit of a separate area for the dementia unit. Otherwise, staff reported spending time looking for wandering residents they feared were lost in the facility.

We noted that alarm systems were at times loud and obtrusive; in fact, staff disagreed about their actual worth for this reason. A more ideal atmosphere seemed to be one in which residents could be monitored closely, perhaps through a carefully situated nurses' station or some other environmental design, avoiding the need for noisy buzzers.

Some dementia units had additional areas that allowed greater interaction and self-expression of the residents. Examples include the following: a separate room for arts and crafts, a specially designed kitchen for residents (and family members) with such items as a stove with safety devices, a special wanderer's room with items such as drawers to rummage through, a room set aside for artwork of all types including some by the residents themselves, a separate family room where residents and family members could visit in relative privacy, and a validation room used for group therapy. These features required additional space; for that reason, they were most often found in newer and larger facilities. We are unsure of the actual benefits of these features, although they probably improved the aesthetic atmosphere.

Differences in the Therapeutic Environments

To compare settings in terms of their structural qualities, we gathered observational information on all facilities. This process consisted of walking about the unit with a checklist to record specific features. The items on the checklist were then added together to calculate an overall score, the Therapeutic Environment Screening Score (Sloane and Mathew 1990). Differences in the mean scores for the two settings were tested. Finally, using the Therapeutic Environment Score, we compared newly built facilities with older facilities, looking for differences that may be attributed to recent innovations in design.

THE CHECKLIST OF ENVIRONMENTAL FACTORS

During our unit observations, we employed a checklist to rate 12 environmental factors thought to be influential in the care of demented residents. The list was devised with the advice of experts in long-term care. The environmental factors were: (1) shiny or slippery floors; (2) noise, especially loud and distracting noise; (3) odors coming from cleaning fluids; (4) odors coming from bodily excretions; (5) glare from polished surfaces and floors; (6) personal items seen in the residents' rooms; (7) homelike furnishings in public areas; (8) an outdoor area or courtyard accessible to residents; (9) separate rooms or alcoves for small group (and family) interactions; (10) a kitchen available for resident use; (11) a television that was absent or turned off in public areas (television is generally not watched by residents with dementia, and it creates noise and distracts staff); and (12) the overall adequacy of lighting.

Each of these items was rated from 0 to 2. For the first five items (whose presence is undesirable) a rating of 2 meant little to none, a rating of 1 meant a small amount, and a rating of 0 meant a large amount. Because the next two items (personal items and home-like furnishings) are desirable, a rating of 2 was associated with a large amount, a rating of 1 with a small amount, and a rating of 0 with little to none. For the next four items (courtyard accessible, small group areas, kitchen, television turned off), units received a rating of 2 if the item was present and a rating of 0 if it was not. Lastly, overall light level was rated as 2 for units having adequate lighting in all areas, as 1 for those with inadequate lighting in some areas, and 0 for units with inadequate lighting in most or all areas.

Thus higher scores for each factor meant that the surroundings were more therapeutic. A total score incorporating all the factors was also calculated for each site. Table 10.6 lists our findings.

No significant differences were found for 7 of the 12 factors. For shiny or slippery floors, the noise level, an odor from cleaning fluids or bodily excretions, glare on the floors, outdoor areas, and overall light level, differences in the two settings were small and not statistically significant. Five environmental factors, however, were different. These included personal items found in the residents' rooms, homelike furnishings in public areas, areas suitable for small group interaction, a kitchen available for residents' use, and television turned off in public areas. In each of these five areas, dementia units received significantly more favorable ratings than the comparison units (see table 10.6).

In summary, dementia units often demonstrated more sensitivity to design features associated with therapeutic environments for the cognitively impaired than did comparison units studied. That is, these settings tended to include features likely to enhance personalization of an area and the feeling of being in a home and contribute to more interaction among residents, staff, and visitors.

The reason for a lack of difference regarding shiny or slippery floors, glare, noise, odor, and lighting is unclear to us. These may, however, represent factors that are widely accepted characteristics of good nursing home care and are thus generally accepted goals of care. This notion is supported by the fact that, for some factors, such as odors, we noted no problems for most facilities visited. Thus, the lack of differences between settings was due to the near nonexistence of the problem. In the case of noise, glare, and lighting, the opposite may be true. Control was the accepted goal, but problems were more likely. These factors may be more difficult to control. Again our observations in the two settings were similar.

THE THERAPEUTIC ENVIRONMENT SCREENING SCORE

We also calculated an overall score for environmental factors on our checklist and compared mean scores among the settings (Sloane and Mathew 1990). The mean score for dementia units was 16.4, and the mean score for comparison units was 12.0. We found a significant difference in the means for the two settings, with the environment of the dementia units being more therapeutic ($p < .001$). Thus, compared to traditional care settings, dementia units were providing an atmosphere that included environmental characteristics believed to influence and support the well-being of residents with cognitive impairment.

Lastly, we compared the therapeutic environment scores of units that were newer and specifically built as dementia units with those of

TABLE 10.6 Environmental Differences between Settings

Components Examined		Dementia Units (N = 31)	Comparison Units (N = 32)	p
Shiny or slippery floors				
Little/none	(2)ᵃ	58.1%	34.4%	.12
Small amount	(1)	35.5	46.9	
Large amount	(0)	18.8	6.5	
Loud distracting noise				
Little/none	(2)	51.6	40.6	.68
Small amount	(1)	35.5	43.7	
Large amount	(0)	12.9	15.6	
Odors—cleaning fluids				
Little/none	(2)	90.3	65.6	.06
Small amount	(1)	9.7	31.3	
Large amount	(0)	0	3.1	
Odors—bodily excretions				
Little/none	(2)	89.3	62.5	.13
Small amount	(1)	16.1	34.4	
Large amount	(0)	0	3.1	
Excessive glare				
Little/none	(2)	61.3	50	.12
Small amount	(1)	38.7	37.5	
Large amount	(0)	0	12.5	
Personal items				
Little/none	(2)	29	6.2	.05
Small amount	(1)	51.6	59.4	
Large amount	(0)	19.4	34.4	
Home-like furnishings in public areas				
Little/none	(2)	35.5	16.1	.001
Small amount	(1)	54.8	29.1	
Large amount	(0)	9.7	54.8	
Outdoor courtyard/wandering area accessible to residents				
Yes	(2)	58.1	34.4	.06
No	(0)	41.9	65.6	
Areas suitable for small group interaction				
Yes	(2)	61.3	34.4	.03
No	(0)	38.7	65.6	
Kitchen available for residents' use				
Yes	(2)	31.1	9.7	.04
No	(0)	68.9	90.3	

(continued)

*TABLE 10.6   (Continued)

Components Examined		Dementia Units (N = 31)	Comparison Units (N = 32)	p
Television turned off in public areas				
Yes	(2)	65.5	38.7	.04
No	(0)	34.5	61.3	
Overall light level				
Adequate in all areas	(2)	60	38.7	.18
Inadequate in some areas	(1)	40	58.1	
Inadequate in all areas	(0)	0	3.2	
Mean therapeutic environment score		16.4	12.0	<.001

[a]Numbers in parentheses are points awarded.

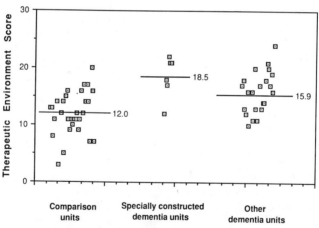

FIGURE 10.1   Therapeutic environment score of 59 nursing home units visited. Reprinted with permission from Sloane, P.D., and Mathew, L.J. The therapeutic environment screening scale. *American Journal of Alzheimer's Care and Related Disorders and Research* 5:22–26, 1990.
Note: Each square denotes one nursing home setting.

older and more established dementia units. We found the mean score of specially constructed units to be 18.5 and the mean score of other dementia units to be 15.9. Figure 10.1 is a plot of the scores of these units.

CONCLUSION

Persons with dementia are too easily forgotten and lost in the traditional nursing home unit. They are unable to verbalize their discontent and bewilderment with their surroundings. They may have problems in communicating simple requests. A specially designed space may help to address these needs.

Dementia units are the result of increased awareness of the impact an environment may have on behavior. Specifically responding to the needs of their residents, they have incorporated several new design features. As documented through our assessment of surroundings, structural differences existed between settings. We are hopeful that, in the future, studies will determine if design innovations such as those we documented enhance everyday living for people with dementing disorders.

References

Calkins, M. P. 1988. *Design for Dementia: Planning Environments for the Elderly and Confused.* Owings Mills, Md.: National Health Publishing.

Cohen, U., Weisman, G., Ray, K., et al. 1988. *Environments for People with Dementia: Design Guide.* Milwaukee: University of Wisconsin.

Coons, D. H. 1985. Alive and well at Wesley Hall. *Quarterly: A Journal of Long-Term Care* 21: 10–14.

Hiatt, L. 1979. The importance of the physical environment. *Nursing Homes,* Sept/Oct., 2–10.

Koff, T. 1988. *New Approaches to Health Care for an Aging Population.* San Francisco: Josey Bass.

Koncelik, J. A. 1979. Human factors and environmental design for the aging: Aspects of physiological change and sensory loss as design criteria. In Byerts, T., Howell, S., and Pastalan, L. (eds.), *Environmental Context of Aging.* New York: Garland STPM.

Moos, R. H., and Lemke, S. 1984. Supportive residential settings for older people. In Altman, I., Lawton, M. P. and Wohlwill, J. M. (eds.), *Elderly People and the Environment.* New York: Plenum.

Sloane, P. D., and Mathew, L. J. 1990. The Therapeutic Environment Screening Scale. *American Journal of Alzheimer's Care and Research* 5: 22–26.

U.S. Congress. Office of Technology Assessment. 1987. *Losing a Million Minds: Confronting the Tragedy of Alzheimer's Disease and Other Dementias.* Washington, D.C.: U.S. Government Printing Office, OTA-BA-323.

11

Designing Specialized Institutional Environments for People with Dementia

LORRAINE G. HIATT

The living environment has four major components: physical, psychological, social, and cultural (Hiatt 1985). These interdependent components must be considered both separately and together in evaluating and developing environments for demented elderly.

Physical attributes are the types of spaces included and their configuration, location, and size; systems like lighting and acoustics, food, and communications; heating, air quality, ventilation, and humidity; and the furniture, objects, and equipment available. In some sense, these are the variables that are most easily measured.

Psychological attributes are images and preferences, such as "home-like," which are defined from the points of view of older people rather than by professionals. For example, people have preferences about seating, about the amount of space they feel comfortable occupying, and about features of that space. These preferences may extend to pattern, color, texture, and other details. Psychological attributes to consider in, for example, bedroom design might be: amount of possessions; where and how possessions are displayed; use of objects to identify space or shape behavior; images produced by the environment, such as security, comfort, neatness or, conversely, institutionalism, confusion, disorder.

Social attributes in dementia care refer to the dynamics involving other persons the demented residents have contact with. Aspects of the social environment include the number of people present; their roles, activities, and characteristics; and their "mix." Sometimes, we "design" the environment simply by taking the person to a space that is populated differently: fewer people, people with different roles, people of different ages, people more or less like her or him.

Cultural attributes refer to the rules and regulations, customs and traditions of a living environment. Nursing homes are communities with cultural attributes. Often strong values and rules are imposed by the staff, such as public display of affection is wrong, or noisiness is punished with isolation. Residents or groups of residents also establish and follow cultural norms independently, however.

What makes designing for people with dementia challenging is the need to integrate all environmental elements into a coherent whole, taking into account the nuances of the illness as expressed in the people you hope to serve. Mandating psychological aspects of the environment or searching for norms is tempting but simplistic. For example, a designer might ask such questions as: How do people with dementia respond to color? What colors work best? People with dementia need traditional (vintage) furniture, right? Or, a casual observer may assume that if someone with dementia cannot answer a direct (but abstract) question such as, "Mr. Bloom, what is your favorite color?" he doesn't care about color.

No single design works for all dementia residents, however. Instead, efforts must be made to understand the individual residents that will be served by the environment, to identify therapeutic goals, and to determine what environmental features best facilitate achieving those goals. This chapter explains the rationale behind design of dementia units and discusses the current state of dementia unit design. Then it provides general principles and more specific guidelines, based on our current state of knowledge for designing responsive environments.

Rationale for Design of Dementia Units

There are several reasons for designing units specifically for people with dementia. These include improvement in resident care outcomes, increased staff efficiency, and reduction in costs. No cognitively impaired person is too far gone to notice and respond to some aspects of their environment. Surroundings can affect mood, encourage or discourage independence, raise or reduce anxiety, stimulate memory, and produce a host of other effects.

IMPROVING OUTCOMES

The environment is an element of treatment that is present 24 hours a day. Its influence on mood, activity, and function can be profound. Over the past decade, increased attention has been given to designing environments specifically for nursing home residents with dementia. With these designs have come opportunities to evaluate their effects on resident outcomes.

Thus, within a few years, we should begin to have enough empirical evidence to discuss the value of particular design choices in terms of measurable resident outcomes. Reduced agitation, reduced physical dependency (which follows cognitive decline), and better quality of sleep are among the resident outcomes that we believe environmental manipulation can produce. Favorable outcomes for staff and families and for the marketability of the unit can be anticipated as well.

MAKING THE JOB EASIER FOR STAFF

Effective facility design can improve staff effectiveness. Nursing assistants and housekeepers often walk several miles a day to provide care. Design features that minimize steps by centralizing storage areas, for example, can increase staff efficiency and boost morale. Resident supervision, medication administration, feeding, bathing, and toileting are some of the many staff functions that can be made easier by facilitative unit design.

Similarly, the size of a unit or subunit can affect patterns of service delivery. If, for example, an efficient staff–resident ratio for nursing assistants is between 1:7 and 1:10 on days, depending on the services provided and the distances involved, perhaps a unit ought to be comprised of two nine-bed entities.

REDUCING COSTS

At one level, we plead for better design because it is part of more humanistic care, creating an enhanced quality of life for nursing home residents and their caregivers. But better design is also more cost-effective design! Sponsors used to overlook suggestions for better design. They assumed that better design would mean significant start-up expenditures, and that limited measurable payback would result for anything beyond safety and low-maintenance choices.

We are now, however, beginning to transform our concern to the opportunity cost. By not designing to suit the needs and capacities of cognitively impaired persons, we may create ongoing costs in labor, maintenance, and staff turnover (Hiatt 1988b).

The question has become, What is the life-cycle cost of effective design for cognitively impaired persons? These life-cycle costs incorporate the one-time capital expenditures of land and physical design features, operational costs or savings, and the costs of consumables. Staff would be in a better position to argue their space, materials, and equipment needs if they could convey requests in terms of overall cost or savings.

If better design reduces steps, turnover of staff, and absenteeism, for example, then it helps staff and can be expressed in monetary terms. If better design attracts staff, attracts families, and encourages physician or consultant involvement, then it's good for public relations. That, too, is measurable and equates to higher occupancy rates and complete staffing, reducing the need for expensive substitute personnel from outside vendors.

Design Features among Existing Dementia Units

A surprising number of design amenities offered in the name of dementia care are, at best, unrelated to any notions of cognitive function (Hiatt 1985). Some of these features may appeal to family members searching for suitable care environments. Other features appeal to staff, but have little or no therapeutic value for most dementia residents.

Too many facilities equate dementia care residents with the mentally impaired, failing to identify specific characteristics or working from inadequate generalizations about how dementia affects people and their use of environments. Appropriate facility design for dementia requires a detailed knowledge of the impairments produced by Alzheimer's disease in its various stages and manifestations, and of the types of dementia residents the facility plans to serve.

Many facilities develop design amenities for moderately impaired persons and populate the service with mildly impaired residents. Even more common is the failure to consider the needs of severely impaired people as part of the overall design.

Designers and sponsors alike often search for a summary list of design features being used for cognitively impaired persons. The following compilation is based on site visits and surveys of more than 300 institutions. It represents a review of the topics addressed by current design and the varying, even conflicting responses. It is not an endorsement.

To begin with, special units may or may not have special designs. Often no special design feature other than the identifying sign can be found. As we noted in chapter 10, only a minority of current units were specially designed for dementia residents. The majority were modified, often minimally. Frequently the most disorienting feature of traditional units, such as long, monotonous corridors, remains when an existing space is converted into a specialized unit.

Even such basic concepts as size and separation meet varied responses. For example, special units vary in size from tiny (fewer than ten residents) to very large (fifty or more residents). Other so-called dementia units actually are day programs for people who, at night, are integrated with nondemented residents.

In addition, the degree of closure, security, and confinement varies. Some units are locked. Others have closed doors but use some type of alarm system to alert the staff when a resident leaves. Other units are open in an effort to minimize the sense of containment.

Existing units employ a variety of systems to provide security and feedback regarding opening the door. Some doors blare a signal to the person opening them but that allow movement (Cornbleth 1977). Still others automatically lock when a person wearing a special wrist or ankle band approaches. Others remain locked unless some special procedure is performed, such as punching a sequence of numbers into an electronic opener.

Any door that keeps older people from passing or requires special procedures for opening can be a fire hazard. Thus, locked doors require an automatic release mechanism in case of fire.

In some special units the residents are confined to the unit nearly all the time. Other units or clustered rooms segregate people with dementia at night (when sleeping) or in the morning, but use other programs and areas of the building at other times.

The use of restraints also varies. Some units regularly confine many residents with or without clear criteria (but nearly always with some medical order), keep cognitively impaired persons sedated, or use restraining chairs extensively. Other units permit more freedom but use closed doors or electronic devices to help manage wanderers (Snyder et al. 1978; Hiatt 1985; Demitrack and Tourigny, 1989). These wearable technologies provide telemetric information about the location of selected people or, more simply, signal when wearers pass particular points in the building (Rouse et al. 1986).

Notions about color, pattern, wall decoration, and personal possessions also vary. Some units favor bright colors; others use muted or light tones, such as mauve (Hiatt 1980a, 1987a). Some facilities make heavy use of patterns on wall coverings, furniture, and curtains; others tend toward simple, even untreated surfaces. Some units use their walls as museums or galleries, covering them with pictures, memorabilia, displays, or even three-dimensional items specifically for touching; the other extreme is removal of all items from the walls, often in the interest of reducing stimulation or promoting safety. In certain units, the resident rooms contain lots of personal possessions, including lamps, chairs, beds, dressers, curtains, pictures, waste baskets, and mementos; other dementia units are sparse, with few personal possessions present.

Another area of variation is access to outside spaces. Even when there are interesting, accessible outdoor spaces, programs supporting their use may be lacking. In the absence of specific programs, outside areas or "wandering loops" (Calkins 1988) are generally used by a minority of residents. In cold climates, outdoor use is often seasonal, and some facilities have chosen to build an enclosed greenhouse or solarium.

Different approaches to room identification can also be seen (Hiatt 1980b). Some units contain undistinguishable rooms and hallways. Others provide slight differentiation through the use of door jambs painted either in different colors or in varied hues of the same intensity. Others use some type of individualizing device, such as name plates or signs, which may or may not be readable to the resident. Signs can be handmade or manufactured, standardized or individualized. Other units favor some type of picture or object next to the door or in the room that has been selected by staff, the resident, or the family to be a meaningful landmark.

Interior and exterior orientation can be viewed as two extremes of design. The internally oriented unit contains social areas with little outside exposure and often employs "therapeutic corridors," "loops" of corridors, and "front porches" that look out on halls, activity areas, or the nursing station. Such a design orientation focuses attention on the "soap opera" of institutional routines but certainly improves staff's capacity to view and hear the residents. Often the desired effect is diminished because the corridors become filled with the paraphernalia of caregiving (carts, disposal units, buckets, and wheelchairs).

The externally oriented unit, on the other hand, contains a range of interior and outside spaces in an effort to optimize access to views of the outside. Its use of space attempts to provide varying "stages" for activities, ranging from grooming and dining to group work and visiting. In these models, the nursing staff needs to be mobile. Staff are typically out from behind the station, even when the station is centralized.

Finally, varying staff and accessibility of staff can be found on existing units (Silverman 1987; Hiatt 1988b). Since any nursing home unit must serve the staff that function there, the varied staffing approaches of dementia units have implications for design. Some units employ nursing staff, mostly nursing assistants, as primary caregivers, assigning to them a major role in the planning and implementation of activities. Other units are more decentralized, using a team of specialists for activities, social work, and even physical and occupational therapy on site. Decentralization may be singular, providing primarily nursing and meals on the unit, or holistic, providing both direct care and services such as personal laundry (so clothing is not lost) and some hair styling on the unit.

These are the major topics being addressed by current design. A quick review suggests that the features being considered in design lack an overall framework. It is as though the first phase or era of design has focused on protection, on issues of containment, and on the factors of dementia that are disturbing to others: being lost and lacking something to look at or do. As new units are designed, however, they should build upon the experiences of the past decade to create more coherent settings for people with dementia.

General Principles of Appropriate Design for Dementia Residents

Several principles should be considered in planning the design of a dementia unit. These include following and extending good basic design principles, shaping design around intervention, individualization, and producing a continuum of care.

DEMENTIA DESIGN IS AN EXTENSION OF GOOD DESIGN IN GENERAL

Design is beginning to be recognized as important not only in special units or for the mildly impaired, but for people of all degrees of capacity and need. Impairments of intellectual and neurological skills are common among elderly who do not have Alzheimer's disease. Common impairments include slowed speed of response, such as reaction time or capacity to process information and react appropriately, reduced attention span, reduced light reaching the retina, routine forgetfulness (as for names or numbers), and difficulties with abstract reasoning (Ciocon and Potter 1988). Normally, elderly adapt to these changes by shifting what they do and anticipating potential problems.

Design needs to address the full spectrum of facility users, including some visitors and even a few staff. The possibilities range from using lighting appropriate for the diminished perception of the average older adult to designing revolving doors and elevators that accommodate slower reaction times (Pynoos et al. 1989; McFarlane et al. 1989).

As we begin to see design for people with cognitive impairments as an extension of better design for people in general, we will be in a better position to identify the priorities and implement meaningful suggestions regarding design in institutions (Hiatt et al. 1987).

DESIGN SHOULD BE SHAPED AROUND INTERVENTION

Design should facilitate treatment. Thus, we are beginning to work from overall program goals to design an environment that can help achieve those goals. Recent literature on dementia care has begun to publish accounts of proactive and assertive approaches to intervention. Among the goals that can be facilitated by appropriate design are:

- Memory development (Grey and Carroll 1981; Wilson 1987)
- Teaching self-care (Barton et al. 1980)
- Language use and production (Benjamin 1986)
- Continence training (Jirovec 1988; Person and Droessler 1988)
- Teaching wayfinding or orienting (Hanley 1981; Blasch and Hiatt 1983; Weisman 1987)
- Improving follow-through or attention span (Mace 1987)
- Assisting in positioning (Demitrack and Tourigny 1989; Hiatt 1987b, 1987c, 1988a; Wilson and McFarland 1986);
- Exercise (Lampman 1987; Mace 1987; McArthur 1988)
- Sensory stimulation (Corcoran and Barrett 1987; Gwyther 1987; Benjamin 1986; Nolen 1988)
- Improved sleep (Bernick 1988)
- Activity to reduce agitation (Cohen-Mansfield and Billig 1987; Hiatt et al. 1988a)

We are beginning to think in terms of optimizing what the person can still do (or be). As part of that process, we are focusing more on the empathic qualities of dementia, such as what actually bothers or pleases the older person (Gwyther 1987).

Proactive interventions have another quality. They have begun to focus on specific characteristics of the resident (Jorm 1987). Assessment should identify functional and behavioral characteristics of the individual resident, such as mobility, communication, and disruptive behaviors (see chapter 5 for a discussion of resident assessment). In design, such functional impairments and behavior patterns are more important than the stage of disease. This is because, ideally, the environment should be supportive, to regardless of the stage of disease (Folstein et al. 1975). We are beginning to focus on people throughout the institution (and in day programs) rather than confining our concerns to a single unit (Hiatt 1987b, 1987c).

THE DESIGN SHOULD MATCH THE SETTING

No single design, no perfect size, no one model of facility, unit, or approach works in every setting. This is, in part, why it is too soon to develop regulations and codes for dementia design. Unfortunately, some communities and states are formulating design prescriptions or regulations stipulating unit size or features in the absence of a well-founded research base or well-conceptualized outcome goals. Some sponsors have become enamored of dramatic physical features without offering a significant, design-reinforced therapeutic program. Such amenities, which may make favorable first impressions, evolve from sponsors who are not schooled in the nuances of dementia. However, staff members in such settings are likely to become cynical about expenditures on features that fail to improve the basic substance of care for institutionalized older people with dementia and therefore lower facility or unit morale (Hiatt et al. 1987).

Color coding for wayfinding is an example of a design approach that has not proven valuable in practice. Using color to represent locations is too abstract a concept for most dementia residents. Instead, personal possessions and other meaningful or recognizable objects can be much more useful in, say, finding one's room. Cues that match the function (barber poles for a barber shop, aroma for a dining room, clearly identified staff members for a nurses' station) clarify locations better than less representative cues.

We need time to improvise, to study, to compare, and to refine. In addition, we need to be open to many different environmental concepts that might be effective for people with dementia. We and the residents in our nursing homes come from a richly varied society, bringing with us a range of experiences and preferences. Instead of a single formula, there are probably a great variety of viable ways of supporting recall, facilitating pleasure, or providing orientation. For these reasons, building codes that respect variations in program and design, such as the 1990 New York State Health Department code for nursing homes, should be promoted.

CARE MUST BE CONTINUOUS

A full-service program for people with dementia is just that—a program. It is not just an institutional service. It is also not just an adult day care center. The program may be under one roof, or the various parts of it may be linked through sponsorship and cooperative agreements. The objective is to make transition between steps or types of care as easy as possible, minimizing the problems of change for those who need the security of a predictable environment. Just as we have come to think of a continuum of care for older people in other services, the well-organized community or full-service sponsor offers a range of choices or progressions of care.

We are beginning to believe that there may be merit in considering carryover between environments. Just as some people take items on a trip to set up in a hotel room to make it "feel" like home, we may want to consider carryover of objects, actions, and design features, where possible. This may involve continuity in small behavior settings: how items are arranged at the dining table; what personal items are on top of a dresser; how clothing is organized; what places and music together signal exercise or religious services.

It is equally important to recognize that not all people will move from one service (day care) to another (nursing home). Furthermore, there is little reason to segregate residents in adult day care from those in nursing homes if they are both participants in some identifiable, place-specific program.

A full-service program does not discharge residents. It continues to offer stimulation when a person is severely impaired, whether it is the same music, now broadcast softly through a tape recorder or radio, visits from the same program staff, objects from the resident's previous room, and an additional set of soothing tactile experiences.

Steps in Designing an Institutional Environment for People with Dementia

Meaningful design usually emanates from the insights of many different people: staff, family members, peers, designers, and others. The fact that someone has not yet seen a specially designed environment does not necessarily suggest that the person hasn't imagined improvements (Hiatt 1986). Design should therefore be undertaken in consultation with the persons the environment should serve and should be based on the goals it is to serve. The specific steps to be undertaken in designing a dementia unit or other institutional environment for cognitively impaired people are described below.

CLARIFY THE POPULATION

Characterize in functional terms the older people to be served. Determine what levels of physical function, cognitive status, and communication skills are present. Estimate to what extent the unit will serve wanderers and people with other behavioral disorders. For one approach to classifying the needs of various subpopulations of dementia residents in nursing homes, see chapter 5.

In addition, describe staff and visitors, volunteers, and specialists who will use the facility or unit in terms that allow the design to optimize quality or productive time. Descriptions may include present and future expectations.

DEVISE A CONCEPT OF INTERVENTION RELATED TO THE NATURE OF THE PEOPLE BEING SERVED

Mildly impaired people may not need specialized overnight care or extensive nursing procedures. Because their memory losses are often not too advanced, this group of dementia residents often responds well to visual, auditory, and olfactory cuing devices (Gwyther 1987; Mace 1990).

Moderate impairment can refer to a wide range of deficiencies in sensory function, language, activities of daily living, memory for fact and sequence, action, emotion, judgment, and social behavior. A full-service program for moderately impaired people might involve a method of assessing the varied capacities and needs and then tailoring interventions appropriately.

Severe or complex impairment might be defined as the dominance of psychosocial needs by either physical needs or care requirements, or the stage at which the resident is barely conscious or difficult to arouse and has an attention span measured in seconds rather than minutes (Nolen 1988). An example of dominating physical needs might be severe bowel and bladder incontinence, physical rigidity, concomitant difficulties responding to human voices, or behavioral conditions warranting vigilance, such as perpetual violence, self-damaging behavior, or choking.

LOOK AT EXISTING FACILITY, EQUIPMENT, AND RESIDENTS

Building a new unit is an option not available to all nursing homes. If you plan on converting or modifying an existing space, carefully evaluate it. Ask questions like:

- What hazards present themselves?
- What spaces lend themselves to freedom of movement, inside and out?
- Are areas appropriate for small groups available?
- What facilities lend themselves to group programs?
- Is there space for a specially designated program room containing items capable of being used, touched, and referred to or objects that are meaningful to the participants?
- How might elements of the proposed program be implemented throughout the facility, perhaps even for people who are too severely impaired to benefit from group work but are capable of responding to simple stimuli like soft textures, warmth (e.g., slippers), familiar foods, vistas, or even the comforts of a relaxing bath?
- Are there redundant stimuli, repetitious rooms, or arrangements that make wayfinding unduly complicated? If so, how might redundancy be eliminated without making the unit look like a circus?

- How can rooms and corridors be individualized?
- Are there commonalities among the residents, their heritage, geographic roots, community interests, or tastes that might be expressed simply, safely, and symbolically in the decor? Such elements might involve spaces, such as gathering around the hearth, the dining room or kitchen table, or at a "local coffee shop." They may also involve objects, patterns, or themes. Such elements may help distinguish one facility and set of programs from another, especially if these same features are used as the backdrop or cue for group discussions, informal visiting, or conversation.

DRAFT A CONCEPT OF THE PROGRAM

Next, seek to determine what each department will offer to the target population of your program. Define food service and nursing assistants' priorities. Clarify the roles of therapeutic recreation staff and of volunteers. Identify the direct care as well as family interaction responsibilities of social workers and clergy. If a range of dementia residents will be served, list what each group of staff or each department will do for people with varying degrees of impairment (mild, moderate, complex).

If departments such as housekeeping, maintenance, purchasing, or security are to have special assignments that deviate from traditional patterns of service, they need to be engaged in the planning or have their needs represented. Knowing what will be offered by whom is important in allocating scarce resources to the appropriate design amenities.

In developing a program concept, the many special issues and questions of dementia care must be addressed. For example, what interventions can be developed for people with a diminished attention span? How can people who are inattentive for a full mealtime be approached? Will facilities for offering meals or snacks be needed for a longer period of the day? Are there features contributing to inattentiveness that must be managed through architectural or administrative means? Similarly, if unit residents will be mildly impaired and mobile, how might landmarks and distinguishable features be used to support wayfinding? Do design features such as noise, traffic or clutter, lack of staff contact (due to distances), or lack of human contact and texture exacerbate agitation?

In years past, the tendency was to immobilize cognitively impaired people and remove objects from their personal space. Now the approach is to provide increased stimulation while reducing stress (Mace 1990). Both immobility and lack of objects are currently being reconsidered because they seem to worsen rather than alleviate physical decline (Hiatt 1988a). For example, many people with mild or moderate cognitive impairment are far better candidates for exercise and movement than we once thought. The extent of the exercise and the equipment used may need alteration, and medical consultation should be sought. Exercises can be done standing or from a chair, as part of daily routines or as special activities.

Particular planning should be given to the organization's approach to concurrent impairments, such as incontinence and decline in mobility or balance. Cognitively impaired persons have benefited from routines and interventions that optimize toileting and maintain skin care. Some of these require policy decisions, perhaps because of difficulties within the existing design. Others suggest the need for new amenities, spaces, or facilities to accommodate a meaningful program.

Put another way, the institution of the future ought to be a place that can be superior to the household or home in offering a safe setting that reinforces the routines and activities that hold appeal for the individual or that benefit higher functioning and well-being.

DEVELOP SPECIFIC PLANS FOR WANDERING AND RESTRAINTS

Determine whether movement will be curtailed and whether and how restraints are to be used, and use these decisions in setting environmental priorities. Consider the many forms of wandering as you plan. For example, you may want to handle idle pacing differently from rummaging (Hiatt 1985); each may need appropriate and interesting places. One facility developed an energy outlet room that allowed both pacing and rummaging (in specially selected cupboards, drawers, a rolltop desk, and closets) in one program center (Hiatt et al. 1987). Prevention of attempts to leave, especially in emotionally extreme states, may require more than one intervention approach: singing and exercise to deal with the emotive energy, actual walks or wheelings about or outings to deal with the sense of confinement, and a security system.

A full-service program to deal with wandering would start with an analysis of clinical care: medications, food-medication-exercise interactions, and methods of dealing with agitation and stress. Places to explore may be one aspect of a fuller program of services appropriately offered to present residents.

What will you be doing regarding physical restraints, either body holders or geriatric wheelchairs? A number of facilities have planned a series of safety features from perimeter controls (Rouse et al. 1986) to fire-rated carpeting to absorb falls in order to minimize body holders and geri-chairs, at least for newly admitted residents (Demitrack and Tourigny 1989; Folmar and Wilson 1989).

Providing the least restrictive alternative usually has several design implications. To avoid the image of confinement yet minimize the likelihood of dangerous elopement to highways, ravines, or other outside hazards, the site needs a combination of artificial and natural features

(Hiatt 1980c). Supervised and unsupervised exits may require signal systems, preferably those that sound pleasant (and do not drive the resident through the open door as a means of escaping the annoying sound). Certain supply areas need separation, doors, or camouflage to minimize their attractiveness. Chairs need to be fitted to people—that is, sized so that restraints are not needed to keep the older person from sliding within or out of the chair. And floors may require safety treatments. Soft yet durable surfaces, including carpeting or other fabricated alternatives, can provide a safety net should a fall occur.

Restraint-free environments do not occur without careful examination of the treatment regimen, the unit design, and the products available. When staff members are not given environmental supports, they often resort to restraints out of concern about their capacity to monitor residents effectively.

DEVELOP SCHEDULES AND ASSESS MULTI-USE SPACES

Once policies and an initial list of space needs are crafted, it is time to get realistic about what can be accomplished, given all of the other services the nursing home performs. To avoid overprogramming and overdesign, translate the preceding steps into schedules for each group of residents and staff. Who does what, when, and with whom? How many people will really be involved? Where?

Each individual department and each subunit within a department may start its schedule in terms of required duties. Another approach is to build the schedule from the perspective of the residents' day, fitting in medications, passes, bedmaking, floor cleaning, bathing, trips to and from the dining room, toileting, charting, and staff meetings, trips off the unit, and elevator competition. Typically, the schedule becomes most complicated around morning care and breakfast delivery.

The best prototypical schedules start with a day and work up to a week, a month, and a season. Will the program follow people throughout the day? Will it respond to those who are up or restless at night? And, in each case, what do you want the environment to do to support the concepts of intervention?

The responses need to be detailed, preferably in written form. Include the unpredictable items, behaviors that occur on units at any time: move-ins, deaths, falls, wandering, agitation, and disagreements. Identify who will be responsible for wandering, for example, on a daily basis. Try to determine how the space and design will operate when different numbers of staff are present. (For example, does the wandering garden make sense at night?)

Scheduling promotes realism about the program. It helps you to avoid counting the same person in three places at once, to estimate walking distances and waiting times correctly, and to clarify who and what needs to be where and when in order to have a relatively smooth operation.

The schedule may help to suggest ways of getting staff to perform interactions, combining such activities as participatory grooming, exercise, toilet training, fresh air, informal memory development, and so on. The schedule may also suggest aspects of the service that are labor intensive or explain why one department waits for residents while another is overburdened. The schedule may suggest advantages for locating some staff on a unit or designing dining spaces separate from those for program.

The schedule enables social services or others who explain the unit to prospective families or residents to know what can be seen when. It also helps them identify design features that show off a program, even though the grooming center, meandering path, small group discussions, energy outlet program, or sleep inducing evening activities may not be happening during the visit.

ORIENT DECISION MAKERS TO THE RESIDENTS, THE PROGRAM, AND DESIGN ISSUES

In both new construction and replacement or refurbishment projects, all the players need to understand the concepts. This includes the owner or board, the administration, direct care providers, the design team, the contractors, as well as those involved in funding. The involvement with detail may vary, but having one set of expectations and one vision is critical to implementation.

When programs are developed in existing, operational facilities, there is a particular danger that planning will be done independently of the units or people who will be essential in implementation. The housekeepers need to understand the value of possessions for cueing or jogging memory and their significance in identifying the resident's own territory or room. The purchasing agents need to understand how each product is to be used and by whom. They need examples and criteria for product evaluation. They may also need help in terms of information sources, such as colleagues, trade shows, and nursing or long-term-care magazines.

Interior designers or those fulfilling that role must understand program goals and decisions, so that they can appreciate and use them. In dementia care, we've come to learn that if it works, it's probably worth pursuing. Typically, if design is based on the residents' needs, the building begins to "look right" and to appeal to families. Families seldom object to design that works, especially when modifications or choices have been explained (both in person and in writing) along the way.

Maintenance workers need to understand the devastating effects of noisy mowers, construction, hammering, and other activities. The more they can understand and work within a schedule, the less noxious these activities may seem. When maintenance staff understand the significance of fresh air, air movement, and a well-repaired unit to residents with dementia, who are highly vulnerable to stagnant air and a poorly functioning environment, they, too, are part of the intervention team.

Similarly, environmental services staff need insights into how to store products to minimize the curiosity of residents, and into the significance of returning clothing to a person who defines herself and her environment by a familiar dress, slip, or robe.

Furniture arrangements should support the programs and services. Where space is scarce it may be necessary to remove little-used items. If needed, outside storage can be rented to make more space available to residents, especially if the program is defined around group work and freedom of exploration.

Once staff of all supporting departments are oriented to the concepts, they can often offer wonderful details and suggestions for expanding the concept without necessarily incurring additional cost.

PLAN FOR PROGRAM CHANGE THROUGH DESIGN FLEXIBILITY

Every planning group encounters some people who speak to the alternatives. What if people aren't as mobile as expected? What if the home identifies more than 16 people who would benefit from proposed design amenities?

Often, population shifts occur within two or three years after a new unit is begun, due either to changing demand or to aging in place (staff getting attached to mildly or moderately impaired persons and not moving them to other sections of a building when they deteriorate). During planning, functional changes that might occur in subgroups (mild, moderate, complex/severe) of the projected population should be anticipated, and the facility changes required to accommodate them considered.

It is particularly important to plan when people will leave the program and how they will continue to receive care. Residents, their families, and staff can be best served if your program includes multiple levels (progressive care) within a comprehensive service plan.

ESTIMATE OPERATIONAL COSTS

Develop a management and staffing plan for the program. Look at how the program might change with more or fewer personnel, or at whether it provides in-house day care or a unit-based service. As you study each shift, consider the specific people you would like to have and how much it will take to recruit them, not full-time equivalents.

DECIDE ON SPACE ALLOCATION

What are the most effective staffing patterns for both nursing and nursing assistants (as well as other staff), and how do they affect the size of various units or programs? Units may be large or small with appropriate attention to subdivisions, noise, and staffing (Hiatt et al. 1987; Hiatt 1986, 1987a). Social attributes of environmental design are defined by the actual people present on a given shift at a particular hour, not by the people needed to provide coverage seven days a week.

How large should a unit be? This is a logical question in designing the social environment. Lacking systematic research data, sponsors may glean some understanding from ethnographic and descriptive studies: slightly to moderately cognitively impaired persons appear to function more comfortably when they experience a range of social options (from solitude to small and moderate-sized groups). Preferences for specific numbers of people (the psychological attributes of unit size) vary. Some residents may benefit from occasional or more frequent contact with larger numbers of people. In general, however, dining, sitting, mingling, and activities appear generally most effective in groups of 9 to 12. For some activities, such as eating or engaging in reminiscence groups, even smaller groups may be more effective.

When unit size is being considered in an existing building, a number of issues should be considered. Some of these deal with the ease of creating clusters or subunits and the possibilities for decentralizing services and facilities (Hiatt 1988b). If morning care is sufficiently efficient, staff time can be released for meaningful interventions or for transporting residents to distant programs.

Suppose a sponsor must care for larger numbers of people, a common phenomenon in urban centers, government-sponsored facilities, and some fraternal and religious organizations. Music, exercise, shared formal religious celebrations, and parties seem to accommodate larger numbers of people successfully. On the other hand, a variety of spaces need to be available, in a distribution matching the facility's concept of programming. Or, in the case of facilities that are trying to squeeze a program into an existing building, the program may need to match the realities of space available and population presented.

A sponsor with a significant population of cognitively impaired persons and only large, multifunction spaces needs to consider how to approximate smaller social groupings. Three methods are: reducing the size of groups and scheduling them more frequently; finding some new space, usually by transferring storage off site; and creating a program center or a series of program rooms (Hiatt et al. 1987). Larger areas may be subdivided subtly, by using a combination of furnishings and dividers (even vertical blinds), to allow standing staff to view a larger area than seated residents are aware of. Noise is probably one of the attributes that makes larger programs less successful. When areas are subdivided, acoustics must be managed (Hiatt 1986, 1987a). Any subdivisions should be planned to minimize the visual and auditory sense of crowding.

AVOID COMMON PITFALLS

How does an organization get into design difficulties? Several types of management decision appear to work against the basic objective of offering services appropriate to cognitively impaired persons. Common design pitfalls include jumping to decisions; choosing to serve too small a segment of the dementia population; basing decisions on simplified, highly stereotypical design clichés; and adopting cute, fanciful design features that are unrelated to research on cognition. Dementia program designers can help avoid these pitfalls by following a systematic planning process, as outlined earlier. More specific suggestions for avoiding common design pitfalls are discussed below.

To avoid jumping to inappropriate design decisions, establish a decision-making process that assesses the potential clientele, develops goals, identifies program and staffing plans, and involves all parties who would implement the program. That process has been described in detail earlier in this chapter.

Develop a thorough understanding of the demographics and characteristics of the population to be served. Many theoretical images of older, cognitively impaired persons have little to do with the actual demand for facilities and services. Without proper study, management may design for and seek to serve a clientele that either is not found in institutional settings or exists in fewer numbers than expected. For example, some sponsors insist on placing design emphasis on features for wanderers without considering the fact that wanderers represent only about 11 to 15 percent of a nursing home population (Hiatt 1985); the different types and styles of wandering require different program and design solutions; and nonwanderers may require as much or more attention as wanderers (Snyder et al. 1978).

Many sponsors seek to develop dementia care programs and facilities that are limited to mobile residents, those who ambulate without assistance. However, a growing body of research suggests that without appropriate interventions (and even with them), the population of wheelchair users among mild and moderately impaired persons is significant. Thus, the environment may need to respond to changes in the mobility of residents. Similarly, as home care and day treatment programs expand in some areas, the demand for institutional facilities for mildly impaired persons can be expected to drop off.

To avoid such problems, data from actual people should be used to conceptualize the target clientele for a program. Estimate the prevalence of the types of problems you wish to serve, using as sources published data, real charts, and real evaluations. Then develop a program that responds to different manifestations of impairment as well as to different severities of impairment (including mobility).

Intervention programs and design need to be adjusted to the nature of the residents. This means that even organizations of moderate size (100 beds or less) may need to have a variety of options rather than one method of responding to all residents with dementing illness.

Free yourself from highly publicized, stereotypical design clichés. I have encountered government officials, designers, sponsors, administrators, nurses and other clinicians with simplistic notions of what design features are critical. One of the best current examples is the wandering loop. If it has merit, the wandering loop is valuable only when another design configuration would be repetitive; it certainly is not likely to help demented residents understand or feel oriented within their living environment. A wandering loop is not a program, but one of many possible ways of encouraging movement. When design becomes fixed or set before the sponsor develops experience with the residents, good money is often invested without real improvement in the daily care available to cognitively impaired people.

The best way to avoid nontherapeutic and costly design clichés is to approach unit design in several stages. Identify your goals, such as protecting those who are ambulatory and who lack judgment from such risks as leaving a secure area (inside or outside) and encountering traffic or hazardous elements. By taking the time to develop a program concept (much like a curriculum and daily schedule), it may be possible to match design features with program emphasis. If the program is to emphasize self-care, activities of daily living, grooming, and muscle tone and relaxation, for example, then the spaces and tools associated with those services should take priority over certain outside features or even fancy signs. The sponsor may eventually do it all (even the wandering garden and sign system). The question is one of how scarce resources are meaningfully spent and available as experience with the program proceeds.

Brightly colored halls or door jambs, bubbling columns of colored water, miniature street fairs, murals of tropical rain forests, supergraphics of arrows or footprints leading to a dining room, beanbag chairs—all of these have been provided in the name of design for cognitively impaired persons. Such elements frequently are unsuccessful because they require abstract reasoning abilities, nontraditional design preferences, or judgment skills that most dementia residents lack. Normatively speaking, these elements may help get an organization started, but they too often become symbolic of the trivial pursuit of elusive memories.

Color coding can, of course, work for the nondemented. After all, we paint our door or mark a key to differentiate it from another one. Unfortunately, however, such cuing systems generally require both memory and abstract reasoning skills, abilities that are among the earliest to become impaired in Alzheimer's disease. Thus, color coding and many similar fanciful design features tend to overestimate the abstract reasoning abilities of dementia residents in nursing homes and underestimate the complexity of information such features present.

We need to differentiate between what may affect people for a first impression and what will be used every day. How many people have historically relied on door jamb color to locate a room? What does bubbling water (or similar neon signs) have to do with eliciting memory unless it is related to some cultural, work, or geographic experience?

The best way to avoid design features that are not useful therapeutically is to look for actual evidence that each design feature works. As sources, use both publications (with data) and observation (in actual visits or documentary films). Be tough on designers, gerontologists, or others who offer a quick fix for the full range of people with cognitive impairments.

Research Needs

Much remains to be learned about designing and using environments in managing dementia. Hopefully, future research will help us find better answers to questions such as how to deal with elderly people in both large-scale and smaller environments and with different life experiences.

We need research that clarifies spatial issues, systems (communications and security, lighting and sound), wayfinding, color responsiveness, reaction to patterns, usefulness of objects as stimuli for memory and activities, role of music and art, and the relative hierarchy of stimuli dementia residents at different stages are able to absorb. These are some of the things that go into households, day care centers, and an array of institutional environments.

We also need research on the numbers of people that residents with different levels of impairment and different life experiences can tolerate.

We need this information to plan groups and to plan units, to provide appropriate settings and activities for a full and varied resident day, and to offer families better choices.

At the microenvironmental level, we need to develop a better understanding of what stimuli to incorporate into which efforts for what type of resident. For example, one person with moderate impairment for facts or sequences may still respond to visual stimuli recalling family life, especially if family life was significant. Another person with moderate impairment may respond better to stimuli introduced by olfactory cues, as fresh breakfast breads and beverages may cue mealtime. A multitude of pictures may confuse one person while providing memory stimulation and room identification for another.

Finally, we should work to develop a model of responsiveness to stimuli. A better understanding of the hierarchy of stimuli to which the person can respond would also provide clues to what evokes sensory overload. Sensory overload appears to occur when stimuli compete for scarce attention, or when too many stimuli penetrate awareness. By understanding what stimuli the person responds to, we would avoid unnecessarily reducing environments to barrenness or sterility in the name of effectively meeting stimulus needs (Lawton 1980).

Reflection

One of the great misconceptions regarding serving cognitively impaired persons is that we know what we are doing. Another is that we know that what we are doing will produce benefits. At some level, we may accept the wisdom of two psychologists: almost anything works because the average traditional nursing facility deprives its dementia residents of both stimuli and program (Kahn and Zarit 1974).

We must develop the programs and interventions—ideally, with some rationale in mind—document them, and hold them for empirical study. The same is true of design. A design for decorative purposes only is likely to discourage staff, take on a cute or annoying appearance, and contribute to a sense of despair about the environment.

We know already about some better ways of doing things. We know that the traditional nursing home has not adequately optimized the capacities of older people. Noxious stimuli draw off precious attention. Inadequate group work spaces complicate service delivery. The lack of personalization and appropriately selected objects minimizes the capacity for cuing. Site selection, building size, safety features, and staffing efficiency all figure into better buildings for cognitively impaired people. However, were buildings simply better designed, they might be in a better position to accommodate cognitively impaired persons.

The key is to recognize that the environment makes a difference, it is part of the program, but the person and the program need to come first. By designing "from the inside out" we are more likely to have environments that suit programs than to find ourselves struggling to minister to the needs of faulty environments while charged with some of the most challenging behaviors known today.

References

Barton, E. M., Baltes, M. M., and Orzech, M. J. 1980. Etiology of dependence in older nursing home residents during morning care: The role of staff behavior. *Journal of Personality and Social Psychology* 38(3):423–31.

Benjamin, B. J. 1986. Using simulation activities to understand elderly aphasic speech disorders. *Gerontology and Geriatrics Education* 6: 17–25.

Bernick, C. 1988. Sleep disturbances in Alzheimer's disease. *American Journal of Alzheimer's Care and Related Disorders Research* 3: 8–11.

Blasch, B., and Hiatt, L. 1983. *Orientation and Wayfinding.* Washington, D.C.: Architectural and Transportation Barriers Compliance Board.

Calkins, M. 1988. *Design for Dementia: Planning Environments for the Elderly and the Confused.* Owings Mills, Md.: National Health Publishing.

Ciocon, J. O., and Potter, J. F. 1988. Age-related changes in human memory: Normal and abnormal. *Geriatrics* 43: 43–48.

Cohen-Mansfield, J., and Billig, N. 1987. Agitated behaviors in the elderly. *Journal of the American Geriatrics Society* 34: 711–27.

Corcoran, M. A., and Barrett, D. 1987. Using sensory integration principles with regressed elderly patients. *Occupational Therapy in Health Care* 4: 119–28.

Cornbleth, T. 1977. Effects of a protected hospital ward area on wandering and nonwandering geriatric patients. *Journal of Gerontology* 32: 573–77.

Demitrack, L., and Tourigny, A. 1989. *Wandering Behavior and Long-Term Care: An Action Guide.* Alexandria, Va.: Foundation of American College of Health Care Administrators.

Folmar, S., and Wilson, H. 1989. Social behavior and physical restraints. *Gerontologist* 29: 650–53.

Folstein, M. F., Folstein, S. E., and McHugh, P. R. 1975. "Mini-mental state": A practical method for grading the cognitive state of patients for the clinician. *Journal of Psychiatric Research* 12: 189–98.

Grey, C., and Carroll, K. 1981. Memory development: An approach to the mentally impaired elderly in the long-term care setting. *International Journal of Aging and Human Development* 13: 15–35.

Gwyther, L. 1987. *Care of Alzheimer's Patients: A Manual for Nursing Home Staff.* Washington, D.C.: American Health Care Association and Alzheimer's Disease and Related Disorders Association.

Hanley, I. 1981. The use of sign posts and active training to modify ward disorientation in elderly patients. *Journal of Behavioral Therapy and Experimental Psychiatry* 12: 241–47.

Hiatt, L. G. 1980a. Color and care. The selection and use of colors in environments for older people. *Nursing Homes* 30: 18–22.

——— 1980b. Disorientation is more than a state of mind. *Nursing Homes* 29: 30–36.

——— 1980c. Moving outside and making it a meaningful experience. *Nursing Homes* 29:34–39.

——— 1985. Understanding the physical environment. *Pride Institute Journal of Long Term Health Care* 4: 12–22.

——— 1986. The environment's role in the total well-being of the older person. In Magan, G. G., and Haught. E. L. (eds.), *Well-Being and the Elderly: An Holistic View.* Washington, D.C.: American Association of Homes for the Aging.

——— 1987a. Designing for the vision and hearing impairments of the elderly. In Regnier, V., and Pynoos, V. (eds.), *Housing the Aged: Design Directives and Policy Considerations.* New York: Elsevier, 341–72.

——— 1987b. Environmental design and mentally impaired older people. In Altman, H. (ed.), *Alzheimer's disease: Problems, prospects and perspectives.* New York: Plenum, 309–20.

——— 1987c. Supportive design for people with memory impairments. In Kalicki, A. (ed.), *Confronting Alzheimer's Disease.* Owings Mills: National Health Publishing/American Association of Homes for the Aging, 138–64.

——— 1988a. Mobility and independence in long-term care: Implications for technology and environmental design. In Lesnoff-Caravaglia, G. (ed.), *Aging in a Technological Society.* New York: Human Sciences.

——— 1988b. Does innovative design exist. *Provider* 14, no. 9: 12–14.

Hiatt, L. G., Merlino, N., and Ronch, J. 1987. *Proceedings: Innovations in Care of the Memory-Impaired Elderly, 11–13 June 1986.* New York: New York State Department of Health/Hunter College.

Jirovec, M. M. 1988. Urine control in patients with chronic degenerative disease. In Altman, H. (ed.), *Alzheimer's Disease: Problems, Prospects, and Perspectives.* New York: Plenum, 235–47.

Jorm, A. F. 1987. *Assessment of Senile Dementia. A Guide to the Understanding of Alzheimer's Disease and Related Disorders.* New York: New York University Press, 88–147.

Kahn, R., and Zarit, S. 1974. Evaluation of mental health programs for the aged. In Davidson, P. O., Clark, F. W., and Hamerlynck, L. A. (eds.), *Evaluation of Mental Health Programs for the Aged.* Champaign, Ill.: Research Press, 223–51.

Lampman, R. M. 1987. Evaluating and prescribing exercise for elderly patients. *Geriatrics* 42: 63–76.

Lawton, M. P. 1980. *The Environment and Aging.* Monterey, Calif.: Brooks and Cole.

Mace, N. L. 1987. Principles of activities for persons with dementia. *Physical and Occupational Therapy in Geriatrics* 5: 13–27.

——— (ed.) 1990. *Dementia Care: Patient, Family, and Community.* Baltimore: Johns Hopkins University Press.

McArthur, M. G. 1988. Exercise therapy for the Alzheimer's patient and caregiver. *American Journal of Alzheimer's Care and Related Disorders Research* 3: 36–39.

McFarlane, G., Bornstein, J., and Proulx, G. 1989. For people with Alzheimer's or other dementias and their caregivers, new technologies help with everyday tasks. *Window on Technology* 6(1): 1–5.

Nolen, N. 1988. Functional skill regression in late-stage dementias. *American Journal of Occupational Therapy* 42: 666–69.

Person, B. D., and Droessler, D. 1988. Continence through nursing care. *Geriatric Nursing* 9: 347–49.

Pynoos, J., Cohen, E., and Lucas, C. 1989. Environmental coping strategies for Alzheimer's caregivers. *American Journal of Alzheimer's Care and Related Disorders and Research* 4: 4–8.

Rouse, D., Griffith, J. D., Trachtman, L. H., and Windfield, D. L. 1986. *Aid for Memory-impaired Older Persons: Wandering Notification*. Research Triangle Park, N.C.: Research Triangle Institute.

Silverman, C. 1987. The resource of environmental design. In Kalicki, A. (ed.), *Confronting Alzheimer's Disease*. Owings Mills, Md.: National Health Publishing.

Snyder, L., Hiatt, L. G., Rupprecht, P., Pyrek, J., and Smith, K. C. 1978. Wandering. *Gerontologist* 18: 273–80.

Weisman, G. 1987. Way-finding and architectural legibility: Design considerations in housing environments for the elderly. In Regnier, V., and Pynoos, J. (eds.), *Housing for the Elderly: Satisfaction and Preference*. New York: Elsevier.

Wilson, A. B., Jr., and McFarland, S. R. 1986. *Wheelchairs: A Prescription Guide*. Charlottesville, Va.: Rehabilitation Press.

Wilson, B. A. 1987. *Rehabilitation of Memory*. New York: Guilford Press.

V

Activities as Therapy

12

Principles of Activity Therapy for People with Dementia

NANCY L. MACE

Therapeutic programs for nursing home residents with dementia have not been extensively researched. A consistent pattern of successful interventions has been found, however, often independently and through trial and error. From existing studies and the experience of caregiving professionals, a coherent picture of the potential impact of therapeutic programs is beginning to emerge.

General Principles of Caregiving for Dementia Unit Residents

Among the general principles of caregiving for this population are the potential to make gains in quality of life as expressed through observed affect and behavior. The most commonly reported gains are improved psychosocial function and reduced problem behaviors. Psychosocial enhancement includes such gains as becoming able to participate in a small group, reduced depression, appearing happy and relaxed, regaining a sense of humor, and having a friend. Problem behaviors such as wandering, agitated outbursts, screaming, requirement for psychoactive medication, sleep disturbances, and hallucinations can also improve with appropriate treatment.

Improvements related to the underlying neurological disease (memory, language, praxis) have not been observed, however (U.S. Congress 1987, in press; Mace 1990a; Coons 1987; Brody et al. 1971; Haugen 1985). Since most dementia residents in long-term care suffer progressive, massive, and irreversible damage to the brain, it is unrealistic to expect gains in cognition.

People with dementia are highly vulnerable to excess disability. Gains occur when excess disability is reduced (Brody et al. 1971; Mace 1990a; Kahn 1965).

People with dementia are highly responsive to their environment, and their responses may be either positive or negative. Programs often observe that severely impaired residents appear particularly sensitive to the impact of daily routines and activities in their environment (Lawton 1981). When a program makes even minor improvements, the participants often show significant gains.

All aspects of the environment affect people with dementia. Therefore, no part of the environment can be ignored or discounted in therapeutic care (Coons 1981). Research has not examined which sections of the environment (staff, family, physical plant, activity program) have greatest impact, but observation indicates that good staff and a strong activity program are the most critical elements (Mace 1990b). Staff behavior and activity programs can produce evidence of improved quality of life even in a bleak physical plant, but the reverse is not true.

Interventions for people with dementia are prosthetic. That is, the intervention must remain in place. This is in contrast to treatment interventions that are withdrawn as the resident improves (Miller 1977).

These principles have significant implications for activity therapists. With the exception of excess disability due to medical causes, the areas of resident life that are most amenable to improvement require the skills of activity and social work professionals. Thus, high-quality activity therapy has emerged as a crucial component of care for dementia residents in nursing homes. This chapter discusses principles of activity therapy, including assessment, program design, selection of activities, and evaluation.

Activities Assessment

A complete assessment of the resident, the activity, and the environment is beyond the scope of this chapter and is well discussed elsewhere (Zgola 1987; Weaverdyck 1990). This chapter provides an overview and gives examples of some of the areas that must be considered.

Assessment of the person and development of a care plan should be carried out in consultation with other staff, particularly the aides. For maximal benefit, planning should consider all activities of the resident's day, including problems in activities of daily living, such as immobility or incontinence. Aides assume new roles as activities of daily living become part of the therapeutic activity plan. Thus, in a successful program the nursing staff, aides, and activities staff share many common goals and actions.

ASSESSMENT OF COGNITIVE LOSSES

Assessment of the resident begins with the assumption that brain damage is largely responsible for limited function and disruptive behavior. Cognitive damage is uneven and varies across residents. Therefore, the assessment seeks to identify the particular areas of cognitive function that are impaired or spared in the individual resident.

Many areas of cognitive function may be lost. The following are examples of areas that should be evaluated.

- Ability to initiate, plan, and sequence. For example, the person may be unable to undertake an activity that interests him.
- Immediate recall and long-term memory. A resident may be able to carry out single steps but unable to carry out a two-step direction, such as "open the drawer and take out the large spoon."
- Performance of well-learned motor tasks. The resident may no longer be able to tie a square knot.
- Spatial perception. A person may have difficulty locating a chair to sit down.
- Recognition of familiar objects. Familiar people may appear to be strangers. The resident may urinate in inappropriate places or attempt to eat inedible things.
- Verbal expression. People who cannot form words cannot ask for help, express pain, or carry out some social activities.
- Understanding of verbal communication. Some dementia residents are unable to comprehend spoken statements. Both expressive and receptive aphasia (described above) may lead to frustration and anger at not being able to communicate.
- Shifting concentration from one topic to another. The person may repeat a word or motion while neglecting other, appropriate behaviors.
- Distractibility. The resident is easily drawn off task. He may fiddle with things, wander off, or become upset in a cluttered setting.

For the resident, these losses often mean constricted social experiences, loss of control over even trivial aspects of the environment, many failures, and few opportunities for pleasure. Such disabilities often contribute to problem behaviors, as efforts to comprehend or act purposefully lead to stress. However, the causes of a given behavior vary from person to person and from time to time. Considerable effort is often required to explain a behavior, and sometimes behavior eludes explanation.

Many nursing home residents have long periods of unstructured time during the day. Because of their cognitive impairments, they are often unable to initiate an activity or even to observe actively. Thus, mental impairment contributes to environmental deprivation.

The activity therapist finds ways to substitute for or to bypass cognitive losses. Planning and sequencing can be done for a person. Distractions can be reduced. Difficulty shifting mental set can be turned to the advantage of the person who enjoys repetitive tasks. Verbal and tactile cues can help to substitute for memory loss and impaired spatial perception. Difficulty focusing and attending may be avoided by changing group size.

IDENTIFICATION OF INDIVIDUAL STRENGTHS

Just as important as identifying losses is a systematic assessment of the capacities and capabilities that remain. Even in the advanced stages of dementia, people often retain the ability to perform and to respond in certain ways. Successful activities capitalize on these remaining abilities.

In general, certain areas of cognitive function are preserved long into the course of dementing illness. These often include a sense of humor (especially when the person is not anxious); ability to enjoy music; old, well-learned motor skills, particularly those with only a few repetitive steps (dusting, sanding, stirring, rocking a baby); large motor skills (walking, pushing a lawn mower); and the ability to follow simple instructions.

PSYCHOSOCIAL ASSESSMENT

Assessment includes an investigation of psychosocial losses. This, too, differs for each person. One issue to explore is the type of personality pattern the person had throughout life. Was she friendly and outgoing? Did she prefer to be alone? Did she tend to manipulate situations?

Seek to identify areas in which the person is no longer able to exert control over her environment or body. Seek to identify to what extent she has lost her sense of body image or identity. Determine what activities are meaningful and what roles are important for her (e.g., spouse, parent, volunteer, busy person, or productive person).

Mood and behavioral disturbances are also important. Withdrawn behavior requires a far different approach than restless hyperactivity. Major behavioral problems, such as agitation or verbal abusiveness, must include activities as part of a comprehensive management plan.

Problem behaviors may give clues to role needs. For example, a person who "takes care" of other residents and one who collects misplaced glasses both give behavioral evidence of basic needs that can be addressed by activities.

People with dementia may also suffer from psychiatric symptoms such as depression, paranoia, hallucinations, irritability, and delusions. Their disabilities may cause them to feel anxious, afraid, depressed, or embarrassed. They are at risk of losing their sense of identity and personal worth.

Psychosocial strengths must also be identified. For example, note carefully such abilities as the capacity to carry out short social interchanges; to enjoy music, pets, or children; to display affection; to respond to reassurance; or to "read" the newspaper.

ASSESSMENT OF THE CAREGIVING ENVIRONMENT

Both the physical environment and the professional caregiver must be assessed. Can the resident hear and see where the task is to be performed? Are distractors present, such as clutter, glare, noise, or human traffic?

What is the ambiance of the setting (rushed and upset, or relaxed and happy)? What nonverbal messages is the caregiver communicating? The caregiver's behavior is vital in setting a mood and ambiance, in encouraging self-esteem and reassurance. Ideally, the setting should provide cues that indicate what activity is appropriate. For example, the bathroom should give easily visible cues regarding its function. If the activity is an afternoon tea, determine whether the setting provides cues such as a tablecloth and a teapot.

Some programs have taken a small group of confused residents with behavioral problems requiring frequent attention to an area off the unit for specialized activities during part of the day (Sawyer and Mendlovitz 1982). They report that this has had a positive impact on participants, other residents, and unit staff.

Principles of Activity Program Design

Based on an assessment of the individual residents and the caregiving environment, activities planning can begin. Development and implementation of a successful program is complex and must be dynamic. Some of the factors to be considered are listed in table 12.1. Some of the most critical factors are discussed below.

TABLE 12.1   Principles of Activities Program Design

Seek activities that achieve these general goals:
    Have meaning for the person
    Reestablish old roles
    Confirm dignity and enhance self-esteem
    Provide pleasure, comfort, or social interchange
Individualize planning
Increase positive stimulation
Accommodate to a loss or diminishment of skills
Use remaining skills and old habits
Minimize distracting stimuli
Avoid reinforcing inadequacy and creating anxiety
Provide an appropriate pace and intensity
Avoid excess stress
Address the entire day
Provide continuity between activities
Fit group size and composition to the task and the residents
    involved
Be predictable yet flexible
Break tasks down into steps
Be aware that repetitive, rhythmic, and outdoor activities are often
    successful
Use activities that are productive ("work")

ADDRESS THE ENTIRE DAY

Activities therapy extends throughout the resident's day and considers all activities. People with dementia need organized, planned activities most of the time, but paced slowly and incorporating normal life routines. Without planned activities many people with dementia will do nothing but sit for much of the day. Because of their illness, thinking, anticipating, undertaking an activity, or even planning vengeance are impossible. They are unable to daydream, plan for the future, or initiate positive behaviors. This mental state may contribute to undesirable behaviors when the person seeks to provide stimulation for himself (scratching, noise making) or tries to carry out an action that to him is purposeful (going home, doing work). Certainly, it contributes to deterioration of self-esteem and purpose. Activity therapy must prevent "boredom" by filling the day with meaningful tasks and yet not tiring or overstressing the person.

Thus, all aspects of the resident's day, not only the traditional "activity" time, must be addressed. The disease so handicaps its victims that a meal, a rest after lunch, or a walk through the grounds is an experience of failure, pain, and frustration unless each aspect is anticipated. Dressing, eating, bathing, and toileting are considered for impact on body image, personal pride, and opportunity for success.

To accomplish this, each activity must be planned in advance, and many are individually planned. This is done in consultation with other staff, particularly the aides, who assume new roles in carrying out many activities. Thus, staff learn to view themselves as enablers, not just caregivers (Coons 1987).

The time after dinner is a period when many residents become restless. Without activities planning, nursing homes often have a tendency to put cognitively impaired residents to bed early. This time period should be planned to provide low-key activities that keep some residents involved until a more normal bed time.

Night waking can also be addressed by the activity plan. When it occurs, toileting, reassurance, relaxation, and companionship may be offered.

PROVIDE POSITIVE STIMULI AND DECREASE STRESS

Eliminating stressors is an essential part of intervention, but it must be coupled with the equally essential task of providing environmental stimulation. The aim of activity therapy is to restore a pattern of daily life that is therapeutic for the cognitively impaired person. Goals might include restoring old roles, supporting social interaction, facilitating mastery of the environment or the body, increasing positive stimuli while reducing noxious stressors, and providing opportunities to enjoy life.

On the other hand, staff may be puzzled because the same residents who are environmentally deprived easily overreact to minor stressors. They become irritable, have outbursts, or cry when they are stressed. Sources of stress include too large a group, too much information at once, human traffic, noise, needing to toilet, or simply not understanding where they are or why. Human more than physical environmental factors are triggers of overreactions to stress. For example, being rushed or being treated as a child or in some other dehumanizing way is a human factor that can lead to intense emotional outbursts.

Residents who sleep are often not being stimulated by activities, or they suffer from delirium. Once delirium is ruled out, the problem should be assessed as an activities problem. There may be too large a group, too long a session, too complex a task, or a task not relevant to the resident's needs. One-to-one involvement (walking with a volunteer, visiting with an aide during dressing, or sitting next to a staff person for extra reassurance) may be the only level of stimulation some residents can tolerate.

It is difficult to anticipate the level of involvement that stimulates the person without triggering an overreaction to stress. Many stressors are idiosyncratic; a mirror may upset one person but be a useful therapeutic tool for others. Resident capability fluctuates over days and hours, making the task more challenging. Many residents, however, give subtle cues that stress is mounting before an outburst occurs.

Overreactions to stress are to be avoided if possible because of the distress they cause the resident, family, and staff. Staff should, therefore, attempt to identify the small, idiosyncratic cues of increasing stress, and withdraw or reduce expectations. One easy rule of thumb is to let a person do for himself until *just before* he shows the first signs of stress.

MEASURE ACTIVITIES BY THEIR EFFECTIVENESS IN MEETING PSYCHOSOCIAL GOALS

Activities should have meaning for the residents, confirm dignity, and enable pleasure. They should not reinforce inadequacy or anxiety. Instead, they should support social interchange, self-esteem, and friendship—those affective norms that dementing illness can take away. People with dementia need a predictable environment, the chance to do something right, and help in maintaining old roles. It is these things that we can sometimes restore for people with dementia.

CHOOSE ACTIVITIES THAT CAPITALIZE ON REMAINING SKILLS AND HAVE A PURPOSE

Tasks that are repetitive, have few steps, are rhythmic, and are part of daily life are often successful. Examples include folding wash, feeding a bird, drying dishes, dusting, and sanding wood. Outdoor activities are appreciated by many residents, as are activities involving pets and children. Confused residents accompanied by volunteers or family members have enjoyed trips to shopping malls, the beach, restaurants, and seasonal parades.

Food preparation activities can be divided up so that each resident carries out one task at his or her level of function. (Sitting and criticizing is participation and may be all that some residents can do.) Participation in food preparation often recalls former roles. The activity's purpose is obvious, and residents can sample the results promptly.

Some activities are less appropriate. Before planning to cut out paper valentines, for example, one might ask: Will the resident perceive the usefulness of this activity? How is this a link to a person's adult life? Might a man think this is childish? What is going to be done with the end product? Will the resident really be proud of it? Is the resident going to have fun? Is she a perfectionist who may be upset by a messy job? Can she see well enough to do the task? Will this activity stimulate group interaction?

Often the success of an activity depends on the way it is done. For example, bingo requires skills people with dementia have often lost and can make them distressed by their nonperformance. However, bingo in a relaxed atmosphere, when it had been an established social activity for the group and when no one is trying to play by the rules, can result in laughter and joking.

BREAK TASKS DOWN TO FIT THE RESIDENT'S LEVEL OF FUNCTION

Tasks can be broken down for a person and presented step by step, or a task can be broken down so that each person in a group carries out one step at her appropriate level. As resident capacity declines, review tasks and break them down into even simpler steps (Weaverdyck 1990).

KEEP GROUPS SMALL AND HOMOGENEOUS

When activities are carried out in groups, the optimum group size is determined by resident capabilities and the nature of the activity. Many residents cannot focus on an activity when the group is too large. Some residents need groups of less than 10, others enjoy the stimulation of 12 to 15. If many residents are dozing or tuning out, the group size is probably too large.

Groups appear most successful when the participants are at a similar ability level. Other programs report that participants with differing levels or causes of dementia complement one another's abilities in the small group.

INDIVIDUALIZE ROLES

When a group task, such as making cookies, is planned, the therapist must think about which residents can do each task, anticipating who is likely to become restless and bored. For afternoon tea one person may put in the tea bags, another carry the cups, another pass the biscuits (with help), and another set out the sugar, all according to varied levels of ability. Active watching (or criticizing) may be an appropriate involvement for some.

PROVIDE CONTINUITY BETWEEN ACTIVITIES

People with dementia need assistance to make the transitions into an activity and to close an activity. If the activity is off the unit, they will also need help reorienting to the unit upon return.

For example, one nursing home was taking a small group of women with dementia off the unit for several hours of well-planned activities. However, the unit staff complained that the women were difficult to manage when they returned. The problem was that no one had thought to reorient them to the unit, the evening schedule, and the staff when they returned. Doing so reassured them that they were indeed back where they were supposed to be and reduced their stress and problem behavior.

Rests or sitting and watching may be part of the day's activity plan. Extensive periods of doing nothing, such as long waits for meals or transport or just sitting create environmental and sensory deprivation. Such daytime inactivity also contributes to sleep problems at night. On the other hand, staff must be flexible and meet observed needs if possible. If a person seems overstressed, she may need time out instead of an activity. If she seems restless when quiet time is planned, a more active pursuit is needed. People with dementia often move and think slowly; the pace of the day should accommodate this, but not with inactivity.

Selecting Individual Activities

An activity program includes many diverse offerings. Individual activities should be selected for their ability to achieve program goals. A wide variety of activities can be appropriate for dementia residents. The next chapter will provide details on activity selection; basic principles are briefly outlined here.

All planned activities should have meaning for the participants. They should confirm dignity, enable pleasure, and enhance self-esteem. Often, activities can also reestablish old roles or support social interchange. They should not reinforce inadequacy or anxiety.

The task under consideration must be carefully assessed. Among the issues are the complexity of the task (setting a table is more complex than peeling a potato), whether it can be simplified by task breakdown, its novelty (using clay is usually novel while sweeping the floor is an old skill), and the number of body parts or objects used. Tasks may also be evaluated for the remaining skills and lost skills they demand. The congruence of the task to the environmental cues and to the resident's past life-style must also be considered.

For example, if making pea soup is being considered, ask yourself which residents can shell peas, wash potatoes, measure water, stir, and give advice. As the fragrant soup cooks, will its purpose be obvious to forgetful people? What will the residents do while the soup is cooking? Will it be ready at a time when residents are able to eat it? How can it be served so that residents are involved but will not burn themselves? Does the activity suggest old roles of a spouse? Does a good bowl of homemade soup give pleasure? Will there be an opportunity for people who can to discuss past experiences, such as how their mothers made soup?

Visits with families should be part of the therapeutic activity plan. Families may be uncertain how to visit with a confused person and will welcome concrete suggestions. Pets and children as visitors are welcomed by nearly all dementia unit residents. Religious and cultural activities are valued links to the past.

The value system this generation of people with dementia bequeathed us was a work ethic: we must find means of supporting these values for our impaired charges. The same values created a funding system that sees activities as an amusing pastime and not as an essential therapy. This must change if we are to reduce resident distress and disruptive behaviors and increase well-being, self-esteem, and pleasure.

Evaluation

Evaluating programs is important for many reasons. It provides the activity therapist and staff with evidence that their efforts are worthwhile; it provides a record of resident change; it provides justification for continuing and perhaps expanding the program; and it supports the advocates who lobby for more appropriate funding for activities therapy.

A brief written log, instead of a more elaborate system, may be best for programs dedicated largely to resident care rather than to research. This written log of each resident's day serves to communicate between shifts, as a reminder of interventions that worked in the past, as a clue to events triggering resident distress, and as a record of evidence of resident psychosocial or behavioral gains. Once a resident has fewer behavioral outbursts, it can be difficult to remember just how impossible she seemed at the outset. As a resident inevitably declines, it is supportive for staff to look back over a log and see how much pleasure they were able to provide him. The log should be used by all staff. If a resident had a bad night, the activity therapist needs to know this. Sometimes a resident may not seem to benefit from activity time, but the evening shift may observe less evidence of stress. Without staff communication, the therapist does not know whether interventions are effective.

For research-oriented dementia units, evaluation can be done in a more systematic manner. Quantifiable evaluation methods include symptom checklists filled out periodically by staff, standardized observations made periodically on the unit by an outsider, and direct measurement of resident mental status periodically using standardized instruments.

Ideally, dementia care is provided by a team, and the team members should contribute to activities evaluation. Quite often an aide observes that the resident was more cheerful and relaxed after an activity— something the therapist might not otherwise know. Evaluation should look for small goals in the area of quality of life, psychosocial function, and small reductions in behavior problems.

Conclusion

Activity therapy plays a primary role in effecting a better quality of life for people with dementia. Those areas of dementia in which change is most likely to occur are within the domain of activity therapy.

Providing this care is challenging. Activity therapists need professional training, the support of the facility, and the cooperation of other staff. Such care can seem beyond the resources of any but the best-endowed facilities, since funding systems have consistently ignored activity therapies as nonessential or nontherapeutic. Further, more people with dementia present with severe and difficult problems, challenging our ability to devise interventions that support dignity or give pleasure. It may indeed seem impossible at times to devise activities dementia residents can focus on.

Despite this, facilities report that even modest activity programs generate change and do so even in people with behavior problems and significant dementia (Mace, 1990b). Dementia-specific units find that, because people with dementia are so reactive to their environment, even minor or inexpensive interventions can be devised that improve quality of life for the residents and satisfaction for the staff and family. Thus, there is no justification for the commonly held view that "nothing can be done for these residents." In fact, their care is beneficial and rewarding.

References

Brody, E. M., Kleban, M., Lawton, M. P., and Silverman, H. A. 1971. Excess disabilities of mentally impaired aged: Impact of individualized treatment. *Gerontologist* 1: 124–33.

Coons, D. 1981. Milieu therapy. In Reichel, W. (ed.), *Topics in Aging and Long-Term Care*. Baltimore: Williams & Wilkins.

——— 1987. Designing a residential care unit for people with dementia. In *Losing a Million Minds: Confronting the Tragedy of Alzheimer's Disease and Other Dementias* Washington, D.C.: Congressional Office of Technology Assessment.

Hall, G. R., and Buckwalter, K. C. 1987. Progressively lowered stress threshold: A conceptual model for care of adults with Alzheimer's disease. *Archives of Psychiatric Nursing* 1: 399–406.

Haugen, D. P. 1985. Behavior of patients with dementia. *Danish Medical Bulletin* 32: 1.

Kahn, R. S. 1965. Comments. In *Proceedings of the York House Institute on the Mentally Impaired Aged*. Philadelphia: Philadelphia Geriatric Center.

Lawton, M. P. 1981. Sensory deprivation and the effect of the environment on management of patients with senile dementia. In Miller, N. and Cohen, G. D. (eds.), *Clinical Aspects of Alzheimer's Disease and Senile Dementia*. New York: Raven Press.

Mace, N. 1990a. Management of behavior problems. In Mace, N. (ed.), *Dementia Care: Patient, Family and Community*. Baltimore: Johns Hopkins University Press.

Mace, N. 1990b. Dementia care units in nursing homes. In Coons, D. (ed.), *Specialized Dementia Care Units*. Baltimore: Johns Hopkins University Press.

Miller, E. 1977. The management of dementia: A review of some possibilities. *British Journal of Clinical Psychology* 16: 77–83.

Sawyer, J. C., and Mendlovitz, A. A. 1982. A management program for ambulatory institutional patients with Alzheimer's disease and related disorders. Paper presented at the annual conference of the Gerontological Society of America.

U.S. Congress. Office of Technology Assessment. 1987. *Losing a Million Minds: Confronting the Tragedy of Alzheimer's Disease and Other Dementias*. Washington, D.C.: Government Printing Office.

———. *The Role of the Federal Government in Special Care Units*. Washington, D.C.: Government Printing Office. In press.

Weaverdyck, S. E. 1990. Intervention-based neuropsychological assessment. In Mace, N. (ed.), *Dementia Care: Patient, Family, and Community*. Baltimore: Johns Hopkins University Press.

Zgola, J. M. 1987. *Doing Things*. Baltimore: Johns Hopkins University Press.

13

Developing a Therapeutic Activities Program in a Dementia Unit

LYNN RITTER

Effective therapeutic activities for someone with Alzheimer's disease must be carefully planned. Initially, information must be gathered from the person and from families, friends, and caregivers. Based on this information, activities can be planned that reflect the person's preferences and ability level.

Assessment

When you first meet someone, it is customary to exchange personal information about families, occupations, hobbies, and interests. This information often makes conversation easier. For example, if a person is a basketball fan, the latest games and scores are appropriate conversation starters. To someone who lived on a farm, the variety of chores and responsibilities associated with that life-style offer numerous topics for discussion. Similarly, someone who was a member of a chorus or orchestra would probably appreciate being invited to attend a musical performance.

Exchanging information is equally appropriate when we meet someone with Alzheimer's disease. Background information can provide a glimpse into the personality of the person for whom you may be planning activity programs.

Good therapeutic activity programming for someone with Alzheimer's disease identifies the person's needs and attempts to meet them through established, familiar pursuits. An example may clarify this statement. Perhaps a new woman on a dementia unit needs social stimulation in order to become more familiar with her new environment. If she had enjoyed baking, she might join a small baking group. By inviting her to participate in an activity she had always enjoyed, the goal of social stimulation can begin to be accomplished.

An initial needs and interests assessment is well worth the effort and time required. Information from the person, family and friends, medical charts, and personal observation can be integrated to produce a foundation of knowledge upon which an activity program can be designed to meet the needs of each resident.

PRIMARY SOURCE: THE RESIDENT

During your initial contacts with a new dementia unit resident, you should gather information directly from the resident. The goals of information gathering from this primary source are to establish trust, to assess verbalization skills, and to learn more about the resident's interests. If the resident's verbalization skills are poor, most information will come from observation of behavior, from facial expressions, or from secondary sources.

When seeking information in a face-to-face interview with a person with Alzheimer's disease, keep the information gathering conversational. This approach is less threatening than direct questions. Questions such as, "Did you do much gardening?" require responses. The person with Alzheimer's disease may know the answer but be unable to express the correct words. If there is difficulty answering, the question should not be pursued. Ask a family member or someone else who would know, if you think the information is important.

In asking a question, the voice tone rises. A person may have lost the ability to understand a question, but the knowledge may remain that a response is necessary. In such situations, the person with Alzheimer's disease may feel obliged to say something to fulfill his conversational responsibility. The response may or may not reflect true feelings, however.

One nonthreatening interview technique is to make general comments and listen for responses. For example, if you offer the comment, "This recipe for oatmeal cookies sounds delicious," a possible response may be, "My mother and I always baked cookies when I was little." That response is logical, and no threatening questions were asked that required a reply. Verification of the validity of the comment could come from another source at another time.

A major point to remember when conversing with someone with a dementing illness is *always* to address that person as an adult. The person may be experiencing changes of abilities but remains an adult and deserves the respect of an adult. Conversation should sound like conversation between adults, not like words between a parent and child. Both choice of words and tone of voice need to be considered. Close your eyes and listen to your own voice and words. Would you be offended if someone were speaking like that to you? This test serves as the best indicator.

An added benefit of providing the opportunity for comments through conversation is the relationship of trust that is fostered. As she feels comfortable with you, a resident may be more apt to join you for other conversations and may begin to participate in various activities. Thus you progress from conversation to nonthreatening activities.

Conversations about music may reveal a history of calling square dances or previous musical talent, or perhaps it brings out the story of meeting a spouse at a community dance. A walk together outdoors may spark conversation about varieties of flowers and trees, previous gardening interests, or memories of a family farm. Gradually, these pieces of information accumulate, helping you to build an individualized program of therapeutic activities.

Personal observation is also a valuable way of learning more about the person. You may find that she enjoys holding and looking at the newspaper or removing dinner plates from the table after a meal. These observations often indicate needs, such as cognitive stimulation in the case of reading the newspaper or household tasks in the second example.

Nonverbal assessment is equally beneficial. Once, for example, a gentleman was observing our preparation of muffins. I handed him the bowl of dry ingredients and a wire whisk and asked him to mix them. He set the bowl on his lap, carefully positioned the whisk between his hands and proceeded to move the whisk in a methodical fashion, completely mixing the dry ingredients. He again displayed the ritual when the liquid ingredients were added, sending a clear message that he was no stranger to this task.

When that incident was related to his daughter and son, they explained that he had worked in a bakery as a young man in Germany. Although the gentleman did not say it, he had nonverbally shared part of this personal history with me. I needed to be alert to the message and gather the details from those who knew. That exchange of information benefited me in programming additional opportunities for bakery-related tasks. It benefited the resident because activity programming could better suit his interests. The daughter and son also benefited from knowing their father retained long-term memories of previous experiences.

The primary source of information, the person himself, is a good starting point for assessing physical abilities and cognitive awareness. Conversing with the person begins to establish a social relationship between you that may set the tone for future interactions.

Table 13.1 provides information that you should look for when assessing someone with Alzheimer's disease for appropriate therapeutic activities.

SECONDARY SOURCES

Family, friends, and the medical chart provide complementary pieces of information about the person with Alzheimer's disease. Spouses can provide information about life-long interests and an employment history. Children may provide insight into current ability levels. Friends may share knowledge about community involvement and hobbies.

The medical chart can shed light on physical health conditions that would cause certain activities to be adjusted. For example, the person with Alzheimer's disease who also suffers from a hearing impairment may not respond appropriately to questions because she cannot hear them, not necessarily because of inability to process the information asked. Facing the person, speaking clearly, and speaking in low tones may assist better communication.

CONCLUSIONS FROM ASSESSMENTS

The needs and interest assessment provides not only information about a person, but also the opportunity to interact directly. From these sources you can begin to determine the capabilities and limitations of the person. Preliminary goals can be formed, stating objectives to be met by the activities chosen.

For example, if someone has the ability to read and enjoys doing so, a conscious effort must be made to provide appropriate reading material so that skill is maintained as long as possible. If someone has enjoyed dancing or gardening through the years, those opportunities need to be offered not only for the therapeutic benefits they provide, but also for the delight of participating in familiar and enjoyable pursuits. Improved upper body range of motion or increased leg strength may be additional benefits derived from dancing.

It bears repeating that all therapeutic activity programs must be planned with a specific purpose, or purposes, in mind. Therapeutic ac-

TABLE 13.1   Key Areas to Assess in Planning Activities

Information	Relevance
Date of birth	Plan birthday celebration
Marital status/anniversary date	Plan anniversary celebration
Names/addresses of children/grandchildren	Plan special events (e.g., storytelling, pet visits) and mailings (holidays, celebrations)
Previous occupation	Conversation starter, subject for reading material (journals, newsletters, magazines)
Religious affiliation	Provide spiritual stimulation
Veteran	Acknowledge on appropriate holidays
Participation in clubs (e.g., garden club, community volunteer)	Provide similar programs (e.g., gardening group, involve in community service project)
Favorite music	Plan music programs using favorites
Previous/current interests (e.g., sailing, needlework, reading)	Provide similar programs (e.g., outing to view sailboats, needlework projects, or appropriate reading material)
Special considerations	Adapt activities accordingly
Hearing impairment	Avoid competing noises, speak in low tones, speak clearly, and carefully explain what is taking place
Vision impairment	Guide hands to task, plan programs using other senses, and carefully explain what activity is taking place
Special diet	Plan baking programs to make appropriate recipes, plan refreshments/snacks to meet special dietary needs, and read recipe books to choose appropriate recipes
Mobility impairment	Escorted walks, lift-equipped van for outings

tivity programs are not simply time fillers or things to keep people occupied. Activities, chosen with care and knowledge, provide worthwhile endeavors that may offer a variety of benefits.

Table 13.2 outlines a variety of purposes and benefits provided by therapeutic activity programs. The list is by no means complete.

Environmental Evaluation

An important aspect of an activities program is the environment in which it takes place. Features such as access to outdoor areas, availability of a sound system, lighting, access to a kitchen, and size of group activity spaces need to be considered when planning activity programs.

A too small area cannot safely accommodate a large group of people who wish to dance. A too large area is not conducive to discussing current events, because the intimate feeling of a small group is lost. It is also likely that competing sounds in a large area will distract participants.

If there is no immediate access to an outdoor area, adaptations in programming are needed to provide the benefits of fresh air and sunlight. If an area has no windows, care is needed to maintain a comfortable level of light, and creativity is needed to prevent a feeling of isolation.

The following sections offer specific aspects of environmental evaluation. You need not address all, but the framework should serve as a starting point. Remember to be thorough, however.

PHYSICAL ENVIRONMENT
Outdoor Area

Determine if you have access to a protected outdoor area for safe gardening, walking (both with an escort and independently), or simply peace and solitude.

Kitchen Area

Look for a kitchen area so that baking and the associated tasks of peeling, sorting, dicing, or mixing can be programmed. Tables or counter space can serve as workable alternatives to an actual kitchen, especially if a water source is nearby. Many tasks in the process of baking require water. In addition, water is necessary for washing hands and cleaning up. Therefore, many baking activities need to be eliminated if no convenient water source exists.

Windows

Windows can provide light, visual stimulation, and a gentle reminder of seasons and weather. You need to be sensitive to the cues provided by views from windows; they may be accurately or incorrectly inter-

TABLE 13.2   Purposes and Benefits of Therapeutic Activity Programs

Cognitive stimulation increases or maintains
    Reading skills
    Writing skills
    Conversation skills
    Counting/sequencing skills
    Identification skills

Sensory stimulation is a variety of stimulation offered to
    Add interest for participants
    Stimulate intact senses, in the case of individual or multiple sensory
        losses
    Decrease chance of sensory fatigue by stimulating more than one sense

Physical stimulation increases or maintains
    Eye–hand coordination
    Range of motion
    Fine motor coordination
    Gross motor coordination
    Endurance
    Balance
    Flexibility
    Spatial awareness
    Kinesthetic awareness
    Strength
    Repeated rhythm patterns
    Vital capacity of lungs

Social stimulation fosters
    Conversation skills
    Cooperation skills
    Feelings of belonging

Spiritual stimulation fosters
    Feelings of peace
    Feelings of comfort
    Feelings of strength

Change of environment (outdoors as well as indoors) provides
    Sunlight
    Fresh air
    Sensory stimulation
    Excitement of experiencing something new
        (Any attempt at a change of environment needs to include familiar,
        trusted escorts and to involve family members, staff, or volunteers.)

Nurturance provides
    Increased feelings of self-esteem
    The human-companion animal bond with pets
    Touch

TABLE 13.2   *(Continued)*

Laughter/having fun fosters
   Increased vital capacity
   Feelings of bonding with others
   Enjoyment of life

preted by residents with dementia. If your program area is not on the ground floor of the building, for example, the cues provided by a window may confuse the viewer. On the other hand, if you only see the sky and your environment is climate controlled, is it important to tell the difference between a rain cloud in July and a snow cloud in January?

Music

Check the availability and quality of a sound system. Music greatly enhances any activity programming plan, often providing a stimulus for long-term memories. Sing-alongs to familiar tunes, dancing, and rhythmic movements are much more enjoyable when music accompanies the activity.

You may choose to eliminate continuous music from a public address system. Such sounds can be easily filtered out by some folk but serve as competing stimulation to many people with Alzheimer's disease, especially in small group conversations or quiet activities.

Floor Plan and Lighting

The size, floor plan and lighting of individual rooms must also be assessed for appropriate use.

Room size may well determine the types of activities that can be successfully programmed. For an area that cannot accommodate large numbers of people, programming may be limited to small group and individual activities. Large windows producing glare and harsh light can be as uncomfortable as dim lighting. Bright areas may be better suited for lively movement and dancing, and more dimly lighted areas for easy-listening music and relaxation.

Plants

Another environmental feature to consider when planning activities is the availability of plants. Plants provide both an aesthetic environment and a potential activity program—gardening. Planting, pruning, and watering are gardening tasks that, many residents with cognitive impairment can perform. Gardening can also provide tactile stimulation, visual stimulation, and a touch of beauty or softness, producing feelings of comfort. Finally, do not overlook the benefit of the feeling of nurturance that comes from tending plants.

Care must be taken, however, to ensure safety. Be aware that any item in an environment might be lifted, moved, or eaten. Avoid poisonous plants, such as dieffenbachia or mistletoe, and injurious plants, such as cacti. Carefully supervise the use of tools.

BUDGET

The budget may well determine certain activity programming choices. The quality of the activity program calendar depends upon the ability of the operating budget to stock and maintain a reasonable amount of supplies. A certain investment must be made to establish and sustain an activity program.

Items to expand programming possibilities may be donated. Perhaps craft projects work well in a particular situation. A list of items needed for the next two or three projects can be distributed to families, friends, and staff members, or even published in a newsletter or community paper. Then items such as yarn, baskets, ribbons, and cookie cutters will find their way from attics to the craft supply cupboard.

Tools for use by men can be collected in the same way. Screwdrivers, screws, wood scraps, and sandpaper are excellent for those who derived pleasure from building something by hand. Perhaps a discarded small appliance can not only satisfy the desire to tinker, but also provide cognitive stimulation in the form of a puzzle to be solved. Care must be taken when using any item that may pose a safety risk, however.

Careful planning is needed when compiling the list for donations. It is vital to make use of donated items in a timely fashion. Good feelings are generated when someone hears a request, donates an item, and then sees it used. Not only is storage time decreased, but future donation is fostered.

Regardless how large the budget, financial constraints always prevent some purchases. It is therefore helpful to maintain a "wish list." Items on it may range from the most basic (a set of mixing bowls for the kitchen) to the seemingly impossible (a lift-equipped van or a player piano). The point is to be ready in the event that funding suddenly becomes available. Responsible planning and budgeting improves the quality of an activity program. Investments should be made with planning as well as creativity.

It is difficult to give a dollar range for an acceptable budget. Each activity professional has different ideas and expertise. Each group of people with Alzheimer's disease differs in abilities and interests. The effectiveness of a therapeutic activity program does not depend upon *how much* is invested but upon *how* investments are made.

TABLE 13.3   Creative Programming Alternatives

Perfect Environment	Next Best Thing
Protected/accessible outdoor area	Escorted walks with staff
Fully equipped kitchen	Microwave oven, countertop burner, countertop oven
Complete sound system	Record player, radio, cassette tape player
Extensive record/tape collection	Public library, garage sales, used record stores, donations
Funds for pet visits (humane society/zoo)	Staff/family involvement of household pets
Accessible outdoor garden	Rooftop garden, portable plant cart, plant stand with grow light

The quality and scope of therapeutic activity programming should not, however, be sacrificed in an effort to cut costs. The budget for activities should be viewed as equally important as the budgets for housekeeping services, dietary operations, nursing staff, marketing, and maintenance operations. Activity programming is an integral part of a total therapeutic approach and must be adequately financed to allow maximum benefit for recipients.

CREATIVE ALTERNATIVES

Because no environment is perfect and no budget is limitless, certain creative approaches may be used when adjusting ideas and resources (see table 13.3).

If there is no access to a protected outdoor area for people to use independently, escorted walks outdoors are an alternative that provides access to sunlight, fresh air, and exercise. They also provide sensory stimulation from a different environment and an opportunity to share that experience.

Lack of a fully equipped kitchen need not eliminate a baking program. Countertop microwave or convection ovens may provide a baking substitute. Portable single and double-burner range units may also provide cooking surfaces. Safety precautions must be observed when using these items.

Indoor plant stands, with or without grow lights, may compensate for the absence of a garden area. If space or safety concerns prohibit the permanent placement of plants, a movable plant cart may be used. Plants can be wheeled into an area or a room for the gardening session and then removed when it is finished. Mobility of the plants permits people who are roombound to be included in an enjoyable activity.

If a sound system complete with turntable, speakers, cassette tape player, and receiver is not in the budget, options are available. A less expensive record or tape player can provide access to countless types of music. A radio is another alternative, but appropriate music may not be playing when you want it.

Perhaps one of the best sources of classical, easy listening, old favorites, sing-alongs, swing, march, ethnic, sacred, seasonal, and popular music is the public library. A wealth of records and tapes may be at your fingertips for the investment only of time. Access to a large volume and variety of music provides great flexibility when planning music programs.

A word needs to be said about television and people with Alzheimer's disease. In general, dementia residents are unable to follow television programs. Thus, television should be restricted to special programs such as seasonal parades, religious programs, musical extravaganzas, or familiar sporting events.

Some television programs may be misinterpreted as real-life encounters and may provoke feelings of agitation or confusion. On the other hand, selected programs, such as the evening news, may have been part of the daily routine and can calm some people.

Care should be taken when using television. Ask if the program is therapeutic for the viewer. Never allow television to serve as an electronic companion or as a distraction for staff. It is all too easy to set a person with Alzheimer's disease in front of a television, turn it on, and walk away. The person may remain seated in front of what may become quite inappropriate viewing matter, such as children's programs or serial programs. Television programming should never replace human interaction.

A videocassette player extends the versatility of viewing by allowing viewing when appropriate to the mood of the viewer, rather than forcing viewing times into the networks' schedule. A videocassette player also expands viewing possibilities. Because feature films are often too long for a single viewing, programs of shorter duration may be more successful.

The type of program chosen should serve a specific purpose. News programs provide cognitive stimulation. Musical productions and parades offer sensory stimulation. Religious programs may yield feelings of peace and satisfaction for the viewer.

Developing a Total Environmental Unit

The most important element of any activities program is the people available to assist in the programming. Staff such as nurses, nursing assistants, and housekeeping personnel need to be educated in the philosophy of therapeutic activity programming. Then they must be allowed time in their schedule of responsibilities to assist in or even initiate programs. The more people available, the greater the scope of the programming and the more beneficial the total unit becomes.

STAFF INVOLVEMENT

In an effective dementia unit, responsibilities are shared by all staff members. Escorting residents from room to room, assisting in basic personal grooming, mopping a floor, serving meals, and feeding when needed are aspects of resident care that should be assumed by all trained staff members. Each staff member may have primary responsibilities, but a coordinated, shared effort is needed to best serve the unit residents.

The nursing profession has traditionally emphasized caring for the total person. This extends beyond the administration of medications and nursing procedures to addressing the person as a human being, recognizing the feelings and emotions of that individual. When the emphasis shifts to paperwork, the human focus can be compromised. Thus, it is important to provide the opportunity for nursing staff to become involved in the delivery of activities.

Nurses generally value their involvement in fun activities with the residents in a dementia unit, such as joining in sing-alongs or science experiments. These activities help establish enjoyable relationships that are not based solely on nursing interventions. If, for example, a nurse usually approaches a resident with a not-so-great-tasting medicine or to take a blood pressure, warm feelings of friendship and trust may not develop. The sharing of a song or a dance allows each person to more enjoy the other.

Nursing assistants also enjoy this variety of involvement with residents, provided they are allotted time to do so without compromising the provision of personal care. Bathing or the morning dressing may not always go well for the nursing assistant and the resident. If that time is followed by a lively session of yarn ball toss or balloon volleyball, everyone's spirits are lifted.

Housekeeping personnel can play an instrumental role in the daily interactions with residents of a dementia unit. Given appropriate information about the disease process, housekeeping personnel are able to interact effectively with residents in their own rooms as well as in group meeting areas. The maintenance of living quarters brings housekeeping personnel into contact with residents on a daily basis. Friendships should be encouraged between all staff in a dementia unit and the folk who live there.

Residents can assist housekeeping personnel with various household tasks. Folding towels, dusting, and sweeping the floor are just some of the daily responsibilities of maintaining a home. Residents should be encouraged to assist in those activities not only to maintain range of arm motion but also to foster feelings of self-worth. Self-esteem can easily decrease if a resident is not permitted to participate in household tasks that were an important part of life.

Think of how you feel when you visit someone who is rushing to finish some last-minute chores. You repeatedly offer to help and are repeatedly thanked but refused. You are told to just sit and relax. That may be enjoyable for an evening. However, if a person is denied the chance to help day after day, the message soon becomes interpreted as, "You are unable to do this task," rather than, "Thank you, but you are a guest and I will do the work."

Sharing activities that are achievable and enjoyable is a wonderful method of establishing friendship and trust. Trust is important, especially for someone with Alzheimer's disease. When the world seems to be constantly changing, and the person lacks the resources to accommodate those changes, trust in another human being can provide a deep sense of comfort.

INVOLVEMENT OF VOLUNTEERS

No matter how many staff are available for assistance in programming, volunteers can be helpful. Students in areas of specialization such as therapeutic recreation, music, art, or dance therapy can add a new dimension to your programming. Such volunteer experiences or internships may mutually benefit student, resident, and activity professional.

The disadvantage of recruiting a student is that a definite course period (usually weeks to months) usually limits commitment. The advantage of student involvement is that students can bring both enthusiasm and an educational background in working with special populations. Often, however, they need additional information about Alzheimer's disease and the specific adaptations they will need to make for activities to be successful.

A variety of nonstudent volunteers can enhance programming. Active or retired school teachers, garden club enthusiasts, music teachers, church groups, or other civic organizations may provide volunteers that will complement an existing activity calendar with new, exciting, and challenging programs.

Volunteer recruitment should involve candor about the abilities and changes in people with Alzheimer's disease. Interventions that allow task success should be stressed. The use of photographs or slides to show real people doing real things (after model release forms from appropriate family members have been secured) can personalize discussions with volunteers, and may reduce some of the mystery as well as the misconceptions about Alzheimer's disease.

GENERAL HOUSEKEEPING

Another consideration is the clutter that can develop in a living situation. For example, a notebook or medical chart is inadvertently left on a tabletop. Baking items such as cinnamon and nutmeg are not put back in the cupboard. Record albums are not replaced in their jackets and remain on a tabletop. Such behavior poses special problems in a dementia unit because items within reach may be moved or carried.

If you notice an item being picked up and carried by one of the residents, ask yourself if it is a problem that the item is being moved. The item may soon be set down in another location and easily returned to its proper place. If carrying the item about poses a potential hazard or the item is costly, gracious interception may be appropriate. The person carrying the item may not give it up willingly, however. An area free of items that need to be protected results, therefore, in less stress and fewer confrontations for all involved.

In planning and doing certain activities, it should be remembered that dementia residents often have trouble processing competing sensory stimulation. A public address system announcing telephone calls, conversations of staff members, the noise of housekeeping tasks such as the movement of laundry carts, and background music from a radio or a record player all provide sensory stimulation. The person with Alzheimer's disease may not, however, be able to filter out competing stimuli, and concentrate on only one. Stimulation quickly becomes noise, and that may quickly become irritating.

One person's music may be another person's noise. People have individual thresholds of tolerance for sound that must be considered when planning activity programs. Appropriate music choices better guarantee enjoyment for the people involved. An initial interest assessment should indicate the types of music enjoyed.

Therapeutic activities, like any stimulation, require the person with Alzheimer's disease to concentrate. The burden of filtering out an onslaught of irrelevant conversations, distracting music, or other competing sources of stimulation should not be placed on the dementia resident. As much as possible, staff should eliminate or decrease environmental influences that can cause processing difficulty. Then the resident's energy can be directed toward participation in the activity, and maximal benefit and pleasure may be enjoyed.

Planning Activities

From the interests assessment and evaluation of the environment, a program of activities that meets the specific needs of the people in the dementia unit should be developed. There must be a specific purpose, or purposes, for selecting each therapeutic activity.

Activities can provide, maintain, or improve cognitive, sensory, or social stimulation; range of motion of a particular body part; fine or gross motor coordination; visual tracking skills or eye-hand coordination; repeated rhythm patterns; reminiscence or long-term memory skills; balance; vital capacity; sequencing abilities; feelings of self-esteem; and pleasure.

Choosing from the smorgasbord of available therapeutic activities requires prioritizing the needs of the person with Alzheimer's disease. Care-planning conferences with other unit staff are the ideal vehicles for addressing goals and priorities.

For example, a woman may have difficulty eating a complete meal because of restlessness. Staff are concerned because she is beginning to lose weight. This problem would be a high priority because of the potential impact on the woman's health. Activity programming could assist by identifying the goal of involving her in the preparation of nutritious snack items and subsequently eating them.

Perhaps a man is losing the ability to walk unescorted and spends more time sitting. Decreased leg strength is a possible result. A goal could be to escort him on walks so that he is offered not only fresh air and companionship but also the opportunity to increase and maintain leg strength.

Figure 13.1 is useful when choosing activities to address specific needs. For example, someone who needs to increase or maintain the ability to balance could benefit from walking, dancing, or sweeping the floor. The single activity of dancing, on the other hand, provides twelve benefits to the participant. Figure 13.1 may be used either to identify benefits from a particular activity, or to select an activity or activities that provide particular benefits.

Activities are not therapies in the clinical sense of the word. When programs are thoughtfully selected, however, they should benefit specific needs of the person with Alzheimer's disease. Different activities serve different purposes, and an activity calendar offering a variety of programs can provide an effective blend of approaches to address a variety of needs.

Figure 13.2 summarizes the activities planning process. As discussed above, planning progresses from meeting a person with Alzheimer's disease, to assessing the person by means of both primary and secondary

Activity	Cognitive stimulation	Sensory stimulation					Social stimulation	Reminiscence	Range of motion (ROM)	Gross motor coordination	Fine motor coordination	Repeated rhythm pattern	Balance	Sequencing	Vital capacity	Feeling of nurturance	Feeling of self-esteem	Visual tracking	Eye-hand coordination	Flexibility
		Tactile	Gustatory	Olfactory	Auditory	Visual														
Balloon volleyball	X	X				X	X		X	X		X						X	X	X
Baking																				
Reading recipe	X					X	X	X									X			
Combining ingredients		X		X		X	X	X	X	X	X									
Make/shape item		X		X		X	X	X	X	X	X	X		X						
Sharing/sampling		X	X	X		X	X	X								X	X			
Bird feeder filling	X	X				X	X	X	X	X	X			X		X			X	
Conversation	X				X		X	X									X			
Craft activities	X	X		X		X	X			X	X		X				X		X	
Current events	X				X	X	X	X												
Dancing																				
Standing	X	X				X	X	X	X	X		X	X	X			X			
Seated	X	X				X	X	X	X	X		X					X			
Escorted excursions																				
Walking		X		X	X	X	X	X		X			X	X	X					
Seated		X		X	X	X	X	X												
Gardening	X	X		X		X	X	X			X					X	X			
Planting		X		X		X										X				
Watering		X		X		X										X	X			
Pruning		X		X		X										X				
Hand massage		X				X											X			
Household tasks																				
Towel folding		X				X	X	X	X	X	X	X		X			X		X	
Floor sweeping		X				X			X	X	X	X	X	X			X		X	X
Washing dishes		X				X	X	X	X	X	X	X		X			X		X	
Dusting		X				X	X	X	X	X		X					X		X	
Laughter					X		X								X					
Manicures		X					X										X			
Pet visitation	X	X		X		X	X	X								X				
Grooming	X	X				X		X	X	X	X			X		X			X	
Holding		X				X		X								X				
Observing						X		X										X		
Science experiments	X	X				X	X				X						X			
Sing-alongs	X				X		X	X							X		X			
Yarn ball toss	X	X				X	X		X	X	X	X						X	X	X

FIGURE 13.1   Activities and their major benefits.

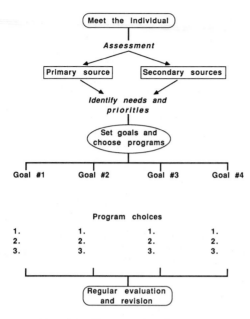

FIGURE 13.2   The activities planning process.

sources, to identifying needs, to setting goals and planning activity approaches to meet those needs, to evaluation.

WORKING TOGETHER FOSTERS POSITIVE FEELINGS

One more benefit from therapeutic activities programming bears mentioning. Working together with people to complete a task fosters positive feelings for all involved. It provides the opportunity not only to share responsibilities but also to combine abilities to achieve a goal. For many people, that is an important aspect of friendship.

Positive feelings about one's self not only enhance self-esteem; they also carry over into positive feelings for others. Communal living even under ideal circumstances requires an adjustment for most people. If residents of a dementia unit can enjoy relationships, each may be able to gain emotional strength from the others.

Positive feelings may also be revealed in enjoyment and laughter. Far too often, the benefits of enjoyment and laughter have been ignored or discounted. We would do well to recognize the value of humor.

Basic Principles of Successful Activities

Since cognitively impaired nursing home residents span a wide range of abilities and interests, individualization and experimentation are important in developing successful activities. Nevertheless, certain basic principles apply: (1) choose adult activities; (2) use a group size that is appropriate for the task and the residents involved; (3) break tasks down into components; (4) combine verbal cues with demonstration; (5) repeat tasks to achieve success; (6) allow active and passive participation; and (7) remove distracting objects and sounds.

CHOOSE AND SIMPLIFY ADULT ACTIVITIES

Choose adult activities and simplify them as necessary. Do not insult intelligence by using an activity that was intended or designed for a juvenile. People with Alzheimer's disease experience changes in abilities but *do not* become childlike. This means they no more enjoy a child's game now than they would have twenty years ago.

Each person needs to be known for the person he or she is. The better you know someone, the more skillfully you will suggest and plan activities. Once again, the library may prove to be a valuable resource for ideas and craft projects, activities, or recipes.

Activity supplies must be selected with care and knowledge. Craft and specialty catalogs and stores abound with choices of items for adults. Often the items are not suitable to use in Alzheimer's disease, however, because the task involved is too complex, the pieces too small, or the picture too intricate. Simplified versions for adults are harder to find. Items designed for children that look as though they were designed for children should be avoided, however.

Some craft objects and items designed for children look like items that an adult would use. For example, finely crafted wooden dominoes with a color on each half, rather than the traditional dots, may be used to match colors or just to work with as the person chooses. The agreeable texture of the wood and the pleasant variety of colors may stimulate the imagination to stack, design, or arrange the pieces in a kaleidoscope of color. There are no rules to follow.

Appropriate parts of certain packaged items can be separated from the parts that are inappropriate. For example, a letter game designed for children may have a juvenile game board and letters in large print on wooden tiles. The game board may be inappropriate but the letters may be ideal for spelling names, spices, days of the week, or flowers. Store the wooden tiles in a separate container and give away or discard the juvenile game board and box. Similarly, if an item suitable to use with adults comes in a box labeled "suitable for ages 2–6," the items can be stored in another container.

CHOOSE AN APPROPRIATE GROUP SIZE

Certain therapeutic activity programs are suited to a particular group size. For ease of distinction, three group sizes are discussed: one-on-one interactions, small groups consisting of two to five people, and large groups consisting of six or more. Keep in mind that for each of these group sizes a responsible person must be close at hand to assist or intervene as necessary.

One-on-One Programs

In one-on-one interactions, a staff member or volunteer works with just one dementia resident in a particular activity. The resident may successfully complete the activity alone or with some assistance. In group activities, like dancing, balloon volleyball, or yarn ball toss, the primary action takes place between the facilitator and one participant. However, that one-to-one interaction can readily shift to include other participants.

Take the example of yarn ball toss. One person may need only an initial cue of "catch" and "toss" at the appropriate times to begin a successful sequence. Another may need a continuous reminder of "catch" and "toss" with each exchange. Still another may need no verbal cues but only the accompanying music to establish the rhythm pattern. Even though yarn ball toss may group several people together at one time, the activity is a one-on-one encounter.

One-on-one activities are particularly important in advanced dementia. By interacting directly with the individual resident, the facilitator can offer cues best suited to her needs and abilities.

Small-Group Programs

Small-group programs are designed to accommodate two to five people plus a facilitator. They require that participants hear and understand readily. A discussion of current events, for example, is only meaningful if the people involved are able to hear and understand.

Grouping more than about six people together makes cognitive activities less than effective. The intimacy of a small group is lost, and the feeling of intimidation increases. In contrast, a small group of people with similar abilities encourages verbal participation. No one wants to risk embarrassment. A person with Alzheimer's disease may be less likely to participate in conversation or discussion if the "audience" is perceived to be large.

Scientific experiments and gardening are two programs well suited for small groups. People observing a scientific experiment should be seated where they can easily see. The experiments I have found most suitable offer both visual appeal and cognitive stimulation. Five or six people are grouped around a table where the necessary items for the experiment have been assembled. Each observer should be allowed the opportunity to participate actively, if possible.

An experiment known as exploding colors, for example, calls for milk to be poured into a shallow pan. One person may be able to assist with that step. Next, food coloring is added to the milk in colorful puddles. If four colors are used, four people can add a color. The final step involves slowly pouring liquid dishwashing detergent down the side of the pan into the milk and food-coloring mixture. The dishwashing liquid breaks the surface tension of the milk, and the colors begin to move and swirl. For those who can understand it, the explanation may be cognitively stimulating. For everyone, it is a chance to experience wonder at our world.

The benefit of a particular program should never be sacrificed simply to include large numbers of participants.

Large-Group Programs

Large-group programs are those involving more than five or six people. Most allow for active as well as passive participation. A visit by pets can be effective in a large group. People are grouped to observe the antics of frolicking pups and kittens or grouped to share the holding or grooming of a small animal. Sing-alongs and use of a parachute (people seated in a circle hold the edges of a colored parachute and move it in wavelike patterns) are also appropriate for large groups. Large-group programs provide sensory and physical stimulation rather than cognitive stimulation.

BREAK DOWN TASKS

Implementation of each activity needs careful thought. Be it baking, gardening, or making a pot of coffee, each activity must be broken down into simple, achievable steps. The statement, "Water the flowers," can be overwhelming to someone with Alzheimer's disease. However, if the task is broken down into steps, success is more likely.

The steps in watering flowers can be broken down to include: (1) picking up the watering can; (2) taking the watering can to the sink; (3) holding the can under the faucet; (4) turning on the water; (5) filling the watering can; (6) turning off the water; (7) removing the watering can; (8) walking to the flowers; (9) pouring water on the flowers; and (10) stopping the pouring of the water.

Depending upon the cognitive ability of the resident, certain steps may be combined. Prompts such as, "Dorothy, will you please fill this watering can?" may be all Dorothy needs to take the can, go to the faucet, turn on the water, and fill the can. If the resident is not able to do the steps in sequence, directions should be given for each part of the task. This method of breaking down tasks into small steps provides a greater chance that each step will be successfully completed.

Another advantage of breaking down a task is that more people can become involved. In the example of baking, one person may have the cognitive ability to read the recipe, another may measure and combine ingredients, yet another may mix the ingredients, and several others may fill muffin cups, shape cookies, or frost cupcakes. Thus, more people participate, more people are successful, and more people have increased feelings of self-esteem and accomplishment from completing, or helping to complete, the task. Additionally, food that is baked with friends tastes best.

COMBINE VERBAL CUES WITH DEMONSTRATION

Accurate verbal cues should be combined with tactile cues and demonstration when directions about a task are given. In tossing a yarn ball a man with Alzheimer's disease probably uses his dominant hand to catch and toss. To exercise his nondominant hand, if he is able to do so, the following approach may be successful.

Stop tossing the yarn ball when it is in your possession. Tell the person, "Harry, use your left hand this time." As you make the statement, touch Harry's left arm. Then resume tossing, perhaps using your nondominant hand, and toss the yarn ball to Harry's left side so that his left hand catches it. This approach combines a clear verbal cue (the spoken request) with a tactile cue (touching the left arm) and adds the toss to the left side of the body to increase the chance that the left hand will respond.

Allow a person who is not familiar with an activity to watch others participate before inviting her to join in. The time spent watching familiarizes the person with the program. Familiarity increases the chance of success. Although you may consider it polite to invite a newcomer to participate, it is better to allow that person time to observe the activity before becoming actively involved.

Statements made to people who are cognitively impaired should be as descriptive and accurate as possible. The comment, "This is for you," is a complete sentence but is vague. A more descriptive statement is, "Jean, this yarn ball is for you to toss." *Who* is identified by saying the name, Jean. *What* is identified by naming the yarn ball. *What to do* is explained in the words, "to toss."

REPEAT A TASK TO ACHIEVE SUCCESS

If you choose an activity that repeats a sequence of steps, such as towel folding, yarn ball toss, capping strawberries, or dancing, allow the person to repeat that task to achieve success. Repetition of a task fosters familiarity, increasing the likelihood of success. The repetition may become tiresome to you if you are actively involved. But be patient; the person with Alzheimer's disease may need additional time to master the task.

ALLOW FOR ACTIVE AND PASSIVE PARTICIPATION

Many activities allow for passive as well as active participation. In the case of balloon volleyball, for example, participants are seated in a circle and the leader stands in the center. The balloon is tapped to one participant several times, providing the opportunity for the psychomotor patterning previously mentioned. Other participants watch and gather information from the demonstration. Shifting to a different person then allows the first person to rest and the next person to participate actively. Alternating periods of active and passive participation provides time to rest and time to work. The time spent in watching allows observers to gain confidence that they, too, may be able to do what they see others doing.

REMOVE DISTRACTING OBJECTS

Before a new activity is introduced, remove objects that may prove distracting to the participants. This is particularly important when food is being served. Suppose a cup of coffee is placed next to a flower pot full of soil. For someone with Alzheimer's disease a decision must be made about what to do with this new item. If a woman just had her hands in the soil gardening, she is likely to place her hands in the cup of coffee.

The burden of this type of decision making should be removed. When fewer judgments must be made, the likelihood of success increases. This provides a greater chance for enhanced self-esteem.

Examples of Activities

The following therapeutic activity program plans provide the purpose, objectives, materials needed, brief descriptions of the activity, and additional comments when necessary for a variety of activities. These suggestions may spark other ideas that better suit the needs of the people you work with.

BAKING AND FOOD PREPARATION

Objectives

- Cognitive stimulation (reading a recipe, identifying ingredients by label, measuring ingredients, and following directions given)
- Sensory stimulation (taste, touch, and smell)
- Social stimulation and cooperation
- Remembrance of positive feelings participants may have enjoyed in their own kitchens

Materials

- Basic kitchen supplies
- Basic food items

Description

A food item is created by following a series of simple steps and is then shared with others. Everyone involved in the food preparation process washes hands before coming in contact with any food item. Each recipe is broken down into several simple steps.

COFFEE HOUR

Objectives

- Social stimulation and refreshments while enjoying musical entertainment
- Cognitive stimulation through recall of words to familiar songs
- Increased lung vital capacity by deeply inhaling and exhaling while singing
- Allowing people of different ability levels to share an enjoyable experience

Materials

- Musical entertainment (live pianist or sing-along records)
- Song sheets for sing-alongs
- Refreshments (coffee/hot chocolate/cookies)

Description

A social gathering for all residents of the unit, coffee hour is a weekly program held in the dining room. Participants share coffee and cookies and enjoy singing along or listening to familiar songs. Participants at coffee hour may be either active (singing along, partaking of refreshments) or passive (resting but being exposed to auditory stimulation).

COLOR DOMINOES
Objectives

- Maintaining or developing visual discrimination
- Maintaining or developing eye-hand coordination
- Maintaining or developing fine motor coordination of hands and fingers and gross motor coordination in arms
- Developing a spirit of cooperation among participants
- Enjoying the feeling of creating a unique pattern of colors

Materials

- Color dominoes: flat wooden blocks measuring an ample $1\frac{1}{2} \times 2\frac{1}{2} \times 1\frac{1}{2}$ inches. The colors include red, yellow, blue, orange, green, purple, and turquoise.
- Work area (large tabletop)
- Participants (passive as well as active)

Description

This colorful game activity provides visual, social, and cognitive stimulations. The blocks are rectangles of wood with a color on both the left and right halves. The objective is to "connect" matching colors continuously until all blocks have been used. The result is a visually appealing and unique arrangement of colors.

CURRENT EVENTS DISCUSSION GROUP
Objectives

- Social stimulation (participants gather together for a common purpose)
- Cognitive stimulation through conversation regarding topics of current interest
- Reminiscence: using current events to recall memories from the past

Materials

- Current newspaper(s)
- Current magazine(s)
- Current events gleaned from radio/television

Description

Local or national events are shared in an interactive group. Participants assemble in a common area so that all can feel involved. A topic is introduced and pertinent facts or background provided. Participants are encouraged to discuss the event or a remembered event. All participants should be encouraged to voice their views and opinions. Noise level should be at a minimum so that discussion is easily heard. Do not read articles. Talk to participants about news items.

DANCING

Objectives

- Social stimulation for both active participants and viewers
- Touch therapy between individuals
- Visual stimulation, including visual tracking to the passive participants as they follow the movements
- Opportunity for active participants either sitting or standing

Materials

- Record player or tape player
- Variety of dance music, chosen with activity and ability level in mind (ideas: waltz, ragtime, polka, swing, even marching music)

Description

The type of music chosen determines the mood of the group. Waltz music is slower; polka music is faster. Once the appropriate music is chosen and playing, participants are asked, by name, if they would like to dance. If so, standing participants move or sway to the music; seated participants are guided by a partner to move their arms in a variety of directions to the music. Thank each participant, by name, for dancing.

EXERCISE

Objectives

- Sensory stimulation through the use of music
- Maintaining or increasing flexibility by putting joints through their range of motion
- Muscle strengthening and cardiovascular fitness
- Promoting bilateral coordination and kinesthetic awareness
- Promoting social interaction in a pleasant, nonthreatening environment

Materials

- Record player or tape player and music (a good variety of music is essential)
- Optional items: rhythm sticks, balls, scarves, parachute

Description

Beginning at the head and working toward the feet, range of motion exercises are used as a warm-up and cool-down. After the warm-up, sing-alongs, ball-handling skills, and rhythmic activities are varied throughout the session to maintain participant interest.

FILLING OUTDOOR BIRD FEEDERS

Objectives

- Fostering a feeling of nurturing living creatures
- Cognitive stimulation of focusing on the task
- Gross and fine motor coordination
- Experiencing the pleasure and visual stimulation of watching birds eat from the feeders hung in the window garden

Materials

- Bird seed
- Bird feeder(s)
- Cup for filling bird feeders

Description

The bird seed container and bird feeders from the garden are assembled indoors with the participants. Demonstration is used initially, followed by resident participation. When filled, the feeders are returned to the outdoor gardens.

Similar Activity

- Feeding caged birds or rabbits

GARDENING

Objectives

- Tactile stimulation of using soil, plants, and water
- Feeling pleasure by nurturing life and growth and stimulating past memories
- Social stimulation, as gardening may be done in a group
- Maintaining or developing cognitive skills by allowing participants the chance to follow directions and to contribute to discussion

Materials

- Plants
- Watering can
- Potting soil

- Gardening tools
- Containers
- Water

Description

Items and participants are assembled. Tasks may include: planting or transplanting plants, filling pots with soil, watering plants, observing new growth, touching or smelling plants, and cleaning the area when the program is completed. This program may involve active as well as passive participation.

MANICURES
Objectives

- Contact comfort with another person
- Well-groomed nails
- Increased feeling of self-esteem from good personal hygiene
- Pleasant one-on-one conversation and social stimulation
- Feeling of relaxation from the massaging effect of having the hands gently stroked

Materials

- Cotton ball
- Nail file
- Cotton swab
- Nail polish remover
- Alcohol foam
- Nail polish

Description

Manicures provide not only smoothly shaped, well-groomed nails, but also a feeling of increased self-esteem and contact comfort. Steps are: (1) remove old nail polish, (2) file nails, (3) clean under fingernail tips, (4) clean under fingernails with alcohol foam, (5) (for women) apply nail polish.

Similar Activity

- Hand or foot washing and massage (with lotion)

PET VISITATION
Objectives

- Sensory stimulation (tactile, visual, and auditory stimulation)

- Reminiscence about previous pets, with the good feelings and pleasant memories that may be evoked
- Developing bonds between humans and companion animals, fostering feelings of tenderness
- Feeling that a contribution is being made to enhance the quality of life for another

Materials

- Available animals (e.g., dogs, cats, birds, rabbits)

Description

Each animal is brought into the area for a temporary visit. Activities with dog: combing, touching, observing, reminiscing, talking to, and playing with. Activities with birds: cleaning cage, observing, reminiscing, listening to sounds. This program may involve active as well as passive participation. In an environment where much contact comfort has been lost, this fulfills a basic human need.

SCIENTIFIC DEMONSTRATION OR EXPERIMENT

Objectives

- Cognitive stimulation, by performing and discussing a scientific experiment
- Sensory stimulation, by choosing demonstrations that excite the five senses
- Social stimulation, by furnishing a reason for people to gather

Materials

- Materials will vary with each demonstration or project

Description

Items for the demonstration are assembled, then the participants gathered. General information is given about the demonstration, the actual demonstration is completed, and a discussion follows.

Examples of topics are: (1) Exploding colors (see above). (2) Water layering—a visually appealing, cognitively stimulating program allowing active participation. Different amounts of salt and various food colorings are added to each of four containers of the same size. A finger is placed on the open end of a clear straw, which is submerged into each container, and a layering effect is achieved. (3) Dancing raisins is a visually stimulating demonstration. A lengthy explanation is required. The program allows active participation at various levels. Baking soda and raisins are added to a container of water. When vinegar is added, it reacts chemically with the baking soda. Bubbles form and the raisins are in continuous motion.

SING-ALONGS

Objectives

- Social stimulation, bringing participants together for a common purpose
- Increasing lung vital capacity through inhaling and exhaling during singing
- Stimulating the long-term memory by singing songs from the past
- Cognitive stimulation, by offering participants the chance to remember words to familiar tunes

Materials

- Record player or tape player
- Records or tapes of sing-along music

Description

After participants are seated, the music is started and all are encouraged to join in the singing. Depending on the music chosen, some participants may dance.

TOWEL FOLDING

Objectives

- Feelings of accomplishment and worth from focusing on a familiar household task
- Cognitive stimulation by focusing on the folding task
- Gross and fine motor coordination

Materials

- Towels
- Wash cloths

NOTE: These items are only used for the purpose of folding.

Description

Unfolded towels are assembled at a table where residents are seated, and the residents are asked to please help fold the towels. To allow for easier concentration on a particular folding pattern, towels of the same size can be grouped together. When the task is completed, the towels are removed from view, unfolded so that they are ready for use again, and stored in a laundry basket.

VAN OUTINGS

Objectives

- Sensory stimulation: visual, auditory, gustatory (when an ice cream stop is made)
- Exposure to the physical and psychological benefits of sunlight and fresh air
- For the resident accompanied by a family member or friends, providing the opportunity for a good visit and the chance to share a new, nonthreatening experience

Materials

- Van and driver

Description

Van outings are scheduled events that allow individuals to experience sights and sounds that were a familiar part of their world of travel and mobility. Road and weather conditions are primary considerations in scheduling.

A WALK OUTDOORS

Objectives

- Weight-bearing exercise and increased cardiovascular strength (for ambulatory residents)
- Exposure to the physical and psychological benefits of fresh air and sunlight
- One-on-one companionship, with conversation
- A change of environment

Materials

- Resident (good walking shoes or wheelchair)
- Escort

Description

The resident and escort must dress appropriately for the weather. The distance is mutually determined. Care must be taken to plan the distance of the walk and to be alert to traffic. Placement of benches at convenient intervals allows for periodic rests.

SPECIAL EVENTS

A word needs to be said about special events, those unique programs that provide a boost of spirit to all involved. In the dementia unit where I work I have planned a fashion show, a talent show, a recreation of *The Wizard of Oz* to commemorate its fiftieth anniversary (complete with "munchkins" from a local day care center and Toto) and a seasonal celebration of winter.

The shows were choreographed, costumed, and staged by a combination of unit staff (including nursing and nursing assistants, housekeeping and office staff), college student volunteers majoring in therapeutic recreation, and even a unit resident who donned top hat, cummerbund, and tails to play Fred Astaire opposite my portrayal of Ginger Rogers.

Special events require vast amounts of energy and creativity, plus cooperation and a modest budget. Our shows provided sensory stimulation through music, costumes, and props; social stimulation for residents, families, and guests; and cognitive stimulation with sing-alongs. They promoted a bonding of spirit that is difficult to describe.

Adapting the Programs

It is a bitter fact of Alzheimer's disease that the illness progresses and causes increasing changes in abilities. A person may lose the ability to read directions in a recipe after a period of time. Therapeutic activity programming must be sensitive to ability changes and adapt to them. To illustrate, two specific activity programs are discussed here for three different ability levels.

Level one is the level of ability in the early stage of the disease. At this stage, the person benefits from verbal cues during the activity program.

Level two is the level of ability of the person who has experienced major difficulties in performing activities of daily living (ADLs). There are also changes in mobility and sensory processing.

Level three is the level of ability in the advanced phase of the disease. The person spends most of each day either in a chair or in bed.

The two program examples used here are baking and giving a manicure.

BAKING

Level One

The tasks involved in baking are numerous and offer a variety of benefits. For the individual who is able, reading a recipe and helping to assemble necessary equipment, measure and combine ingredients offers cognitive stimulation, sensory stimulation, social stimulation, range of arm motion, and gross and fine motor coordination. With subtle prompts such as, "Alice, we need the yellow mixing bowl from the cupboard," the person should be able to complete the task.

The next step could be, "Alice, we need to measure three cups of flour into the yellow bowl." If Alice has the yellow bowl in front of her with the container of flour, a measuring cup, and something to level the flour, she should be successful at completing that step. The prompts are accurate and descriptive, and the area is not cluttered with extraneous stimuli.

Level Two

As time goes on, Alice loses some abilities and may no longer be able to read recipes or move with ease about the kitchen. The activity must adapt to the changes Alice is experiencing. Alice is never forced to accommodate the activity.

At this level, another person may measure into the bowl along with the cinnamon and nutmeg. At this point, Alice is shown the bowl and handed a mixing spoon. She is then approached with the statement, "Alice, this flour needs stirring." The bowl is steadied for Alice, and her hand may or may not need to be guided to the spoon to combine the ingredients. Alice continues to be a part of the event, her role has simply been adapted to match her changing abilities.

Level Three

There may come a time when Alice remains in a chair or in her bed because of further changes in abilities and possibly declining health. Alice may be involved in the baking program by including her in conversations as the tasks are performed. Comments such as, "Alice, we are now combining the flour, the cinnamon, and the nutmeg for our oatmeal cookies," include her in the task. Alice may not be as verbally responsive as she once was, but it is impossible to know exactly what Alice is able to hear and process.

If Alice is in her room, the spices of cinnamon and nutmeg could be taken to her to smell. Again, she is given information necessary to understand the situation. "Alice, I thought you would enjoy the smell of the cinnamon we are adding to the oatmeal cookies we are baking." Perhaps the scent will trigger happy memories of previous baking experiences. If Alice is able, she should be offered one of the freshly baked cookies to complete the experience.

GIVING A MANICURE

A major benefit of giving a manicure is that it provides contact comfort through touch and is similarly performed for a variety of people regardless of their abilities. A complete manicure involves clipping the nails, filing and shaping them, cleaning under the fingernails, and, for women, removing old nail polish and applying a fresh coat. Variables such as time available, acceptance on the part of the resident, and numbers of people to be manicured determine what parts of a manicure are given. If the person is not able to sit comfortably in one place for a complete manicure, it can be given in stages. The clipping and shaping can be done at one time, and cleaning under the fingernails and polishing a short time later.

A manicure promotes not only good personal hygiene, but also provides a feeling of increased self-esteem by enhancing one's appearance. The gentle touching of hands during a manicure is a sign of warmth between two people. It also fosters relaxation and a sense of calm.

A manicure may be the right choice for someone who is unable to sleep. Little preparation is involved, and a manicure at 3:00 A.M. may serve to relax someone so that she is able to sleep. An added benefit is that a manicure is equally appropriate for men and women.

A manicure may also serve as an activity from which a family member may derive great joy and comfort. An investment in a well-stocked manicure kit with cotton balls, nail polish remover, nail clippers, a good nail file, and clear as well as a variety of colorful nail polishes may prove to be valuable for residents as well as family members, to be used night as well as day.

Level One

For someone whose ability levels and verbal skills are good, a manicure may serve as a time for intimate conversation. It may not be necessary to explain the various steps, and conversation may run the range of topics any two friends would discuss.

Level Two

As ability levels change, the amount of conversation may also change. A detailed explanation of each step of the manicure may be necessary to reassure the person with Alzheimer's disease. However, the same steps are followed.

Level Three

The contact between people and the corresponding benefits do not decrease as abilities change. A manicure may be stimulating to a person whose world is limited to what can be experienced from a bed or a chair. In level three, the manicure items may be assembled on an over-the-bed tray so that they can be conveniently positioned near the person having the manicure. Again, it is necessary to explain each step of the procedure accurately. For example, "Roy, I am going to clean under your thumbnail," followed by, "Roy, I am now going to clean under your index fingernail," should give Roy the information necessary to know what you are doing.

You may choose to offer comments about the weather, the news of the day, or any other conversation tidbits during the manicure. You may also choose the comfort of a quiet time shared by friends with no conversation.

The Evaluation and Revision of Activity Programs

Activity assessment, environmental evaluation, staffing considerations, and knowledge of the purposes and benefits of various activity choices are necessary parts of a wise selection of activity programs for people with Alzheimer's disease. However, implementation is not the last step. The programs must be evaluated and often revised.

A particular therapeutic activity program permits reassessment of the ability levels of the people involved. Each time a task is performed, subtle changes may be noted.

For example, a person may have been successful at completing the two-step task of picking up a watering can and pouring water on a pot of flowers. With time, the person may find information difficult to process and may hesitate to initiate any action. When this happens, adjust the task to make it easier. For example, fill the watering can yourself and hand it to the person who is already positioned at the pot of flowers. The flowers receive water, the person is successful, and self-esteem is preserved. Evaluation and revision of therapeutic activities is a constant process.

Flexibility: A Key to Success

Another aspect of successful programming is flexibility. A specific program may be planned, but its implementation may lead to unexpected results. For example, in filling a bird feeder, a resident may become focused on the seeds. She begins separating the distinctive black sunflower seeds from other seeds in the mixture. She does this with great care, concentration, and accuracy. This is not the intent of the activity, but because it serves a worthwhile purpose for the sorter, it is encouraged.

Flexibility is necessary when working with people. Learn to separate your ego from the unpredictability of others. Use your knowledge and creativity to plan the most therapeutic programs and then accept change as inevitable. Change is a part of life. Remember, those around you must deal with change on a much deeper level.

Activities Enhance Visits

As previously mentioned, families and friends should be encouraged to participate in activities. Sharing an experience is enjoyable and enhances the quality of a visit. Becoming involved together in an activity also eliminates the tendency of the visit to deteriorate into a question-and-answer session. The visit is unpleasant for both parties if the resident is bombarded with, "What did you have for lunch?" "When was Aunt Mary last here to visit you?" "Why don't you sit next to me and talk?"

Tasks of gardening, joining in scientific experiments, or singing old, familiar tunes together can foster feelings on the part of family members that an acceptable quality of life exists for the relative with Alzheimer's disease. Visits that foster positive feelings may be repeated more frequently.

Successful participation in activity programs can also serve the valuable lesson of demonstrating the resident's abilities and accomplishments rather than focusing on inabilities and losses. Family members and friends may change their misperceptions when they observe successful completion of activities. Enjoyable time spent together can lead to laughter, the easing of tensions, and an increased pleasure in the relationship.

Support Is Vital to a Successful Program

The previous information, guidelines, and suggestions are only effective when an activities effort is believed in, promoted, and supported. The entire staff needs to understand the progress of Alzheimer's disease and related disorders and the benefits provided by a dementia program with a consistent, caring approach. Education needs to include administrative personnel, medical directors, nursing and nursing assistants, and volunteers, activities, dietary, laundry, housekeeping, maintenance, social services, admissions, and marketing departments. All staff on all shifts should be knowledgeable about dementia and the unit's goals. Not all staff may be directly involved in the unit's operation, but their knowledge is critical to the support and understanding of such a unit. Periodic updates or in-service training may be needed to educate new staff members and remind current staff about the purposes and benefits of such a special unit.

Tremendous energy, commitment, and resources are needed to develop a therapeutic activity program because that program will not be successful unless it is part of an entire environment designed to maximize the success of someone with Alzheimer's disease. Various degrees of commitment result in varying degrees of benefit. A dementia unit, just like any life form, needs to be nurtured, sustained, and allowed to evolve. A program fortunate enough to have nurturance serves its residents well.

References

DeBruin, J. 1980. *Creative, Hands-on Science Experiences Using Free and Inexpensive Materials*. Carthage, Ill.: Good Apple.

Lehane, M. S. 1980. *Science Tricks*. New York: Franklin Watts.

Herbert, D. 1980. *Mr. Wizard's Supermarket Science*. New York: Random House.

Markle, S. 1988. *Science Mini-Mysteries*. New York: Atheneum.

Saul, W., Saul, N., and Alan, R. 1986. *Science Fare*. New York: Harper & Row.

Vowles, A. 1985. *The EDC Book of Amazing Experiments You Can Do at Home*. Tulsa, Okla.: EDC Publishing.

VI

Conclusion

14

The Future Role of Specialized Dementia Care

PHILIP D. SLOANE AND LAURA J. MATHEW

The growth of dementia units in nursing homes has been rapid. Between 1987 and 1989, while conducting a five-state study, we had the opportunity to examine this movement in detail through personal visits and consultation with experts. Since that time, in preparing this manuscript, we have learned more about innovative programs elsewhere and the ideals of professionals working in Alzheimer's care. Based on these activities, we would like to share our overall impressions of the current and future role of dementia units in nursing home care.

Our study results show that dementia units differ from traditional nursing home care. We noted differences in all areas studied—structure, administration, resident population, and provision of care. The smaller size and census of dementia units may be assets in managing the behavioral manifestations of the disease. Specific design features such as small clusters of rooms, visual cues to help identify rooms, conspicuous light switches and door handles, wandering areas, and multiple small common areas are frequently incorporated into these units. While research on the effects of these environmental features is scarce, we believe that certain design elements can engage, orient, and comfort the cognitively impaired.

Administratively, dementia units have lower ratios of residents to staff for all categories of caregiving personnel than traditional nursing homes have. Dementia units notably emphasize activities. In keeping with the concept of specialized care, units tend to select their participants carefully and to train staff to deal with their population.

The resident population on dementia units is clearly at a relatively early stage of disease. They function at a higher level in all activities of daily living, particularly in mobility. However, we noted a developing trend of dementia units to accommodate residents with more advanced disease, often in separate units. In the future the dementia unit concept may be better able to take care of residents at later stages. We also noted that dementia unit residents have more personal resources than their counterparts in traditional settings. A higher proportion of people were private payers, more were married, and the frequency of family visits was higher.

Regarding the actual care provided, we noted significant differences. There was more human interaction on the dementia units, both between residents and staff and among residents. More residents moved about independently, and the use of physical restraints was far lower. Finally, overall medication prescriptions were fewer.

On the other hand, differences were absent in some important areas. Most surprising was the use of chemical restraints, which was no different in the dementia units than in the comparison units.

Another finding was that residents did not differ in measures of mental status. This was less surprising to us, since placement on a dementia unit would not be expected to halt neuronal damage. Finally, the basic issues of hygiene and cleanliness seemed to be addressed in both settings, although dementia units showed slightly more success in resident grooming. Environmental factors such as odor were not substantially different. Thus, nonspecialized care did not equate with a lack of basic care.

The place of physical and chemical restraints in ideal nursing home care has yet to be determined. As we looked carefully at our data on restraint use, it seemed that chemical and physical restraints are used for different reasons. Physical restraints may have a role in providing safety and positioning of certain residents at certain times. Similarly, chemical restraints seem to have a place in treating severe behavioral problems. Use of either physical or chemical restraints may on occasion be in the best interest of the resident. Therefore, units may consider reduction of restraints, rather their elimination, to be the most appropriate goal.

Do specialized units provide better care? Our study data cannot be used to conclude that they do. Because the data report on very different groups of residents, the effects of treatment cannot be separated from those of selection.

It is our impression, however, that demented residents in traditional nursing home settings are easy to overlook. They require constant supervision but rarely ask for it. They are unable to communicate needs and rarely use call bells. They do not make friends with the staff. They lack the attention span to participate in customary activities. Thus, residents with dementia require a more active approach and special attention. We believe that dementia units may provide a setting in which these needs can be met.

Dementia units represent a true innovation in nursing home care, we believe. The diversity and creativity noted in some of our data are expanded upon in chapters 8, 11, 12, and 13, which provide valuable information based on the authors' own wide experiences and those of others with whom they have worked.

This material indicates that new approaches have found success with a population that in the past has been difficult to reach. One can thus regard these chapters as a guide to current thinking on the best practices in specialized dementia care.

Where is the movement headed? We believe that specialization will continue to grow as a feature of long-term care. Dementia units represent only one area of specialization. Already, some homes are experimenting with the notion of serving well-defined clinical populations, such as stroke or patients with skin problems, in segregated areas. Such units should be defined, we believe, on the basis of care need rather than diagnosis. For example, the structured environment of the dementia unit may well serve an elderly person with schizophrenia or mental retardation.

The fact that nursing homes are becoming more specialized poses new challenges for regulatory agencies. Specialized care will be expected to be judged by different standards depending on the population it serves. An early movement already exists toward defining separate standards for dementia units. Reimbursement levels will need to reflect differences in care. Merely continuing case-based approaches such as that of the Resource Utilization Groups (RUGs) fails to account for physical and care environment features that distinguish a specialized unit.

We believe that multiple levels of specialized care for the cognitively impaired within the same nursing home will become common. Such units will reflect the heterogeneity of nursing home residents with these diagnoses by providing separate care areas for people at different stages of impairment. Already a number of larger homes have developed two or more dementia units, with each unit serving a different subgroup. Some of these units will be defined as rehabilitative, others as social, and others as providing terminal (primarily nursing) care. We support this concept because of its potential both for providing a continuum of care and for exploring new treatments.

To further serve their dementia populations, nursing homes will continue to experiment with different approaches to care. Segregated closed units are just one concept. Other approaches include specialized programs that temporarily draw certain residents from a number of areas in a nursing home. For example, one nursing home may bring residents with certain types of feeding problems, or those with agitation, to a separate area for concentrated attention during part of the day. These and similar specialized day programs have the advantage of being available to everyone in a nursing home as needed. They can also be made available to family caregivers in the community.

In addition, dementia units are likely to be in the forefront of developing and testing new technologies that aid in managing their residents. Examples include improved floor surfaces, new types of furniture, and less restrictive ways of positioning residents.

Finally, nursing homes will continue to be faced with the demands of providing high-quality care to a burgeoning population with limited resources. Projections are that the United States nursing home population with dementia may triple by the year 2040. We already face a shortage of health workers, particularly in the nursing field, to care for our elderly. No one is sure how this crisis will be solved.

It is quite possible that the combination of scarce resources, a growing population of demented elderly, and improved capabilities of nursing homes to prolong life will force us to confront a variety of ethical dilemmas. As part of this process, dementia units will have to critically examine the ultimate goals of care for people with Alzheimer's disease and related disorders. Thus, specialized units may be at the forefront not only of new treatments but of deciding whether and when these treatments should be limited.

Finally, we believe that dementia units have had, and will continue to have, a positive effect on the quality of life for all nursing home residents. At the very least, dementia units have taught us that quality of life can be enhanced even in advanced stages of this dreadful disease. They have taught us to evaluate the whole nursing home environment and its effects on the people who live there. They have demonstrated that comfort, pleasure, and dignity can be maintained throughout the course of a dementing illness.

Appendix
The Background, Objectives, and Methods of the Study

LAURA J. MATHEW, PHILIP D. SLOANE, AND JAIKISHAN R. DESAI

The study reported in chapters 2, 3, 4, 6, 7, 9, and 10 was conducted during 1987–1990 under a three-year grant from the Alzheimer's Association. Designed as a cross-sectional descriptive survey of existing dementia units, it sampled for-profit and nonprofit units in five states.

The Objectives of the Study

The study had the following five objectives:

1. *To estimate the number of dementia units operating in the five states of California, New York, North Carolina, Ohio, and Texas.*

Estimates of the number of units in the country were vague. A report by the Office of Technology Assessment in 1987 stated that 150 to 200 units existed (U.S. Congress 1987). Another publication (Wagner 1987) stated that the Hillhaven Corporation would have 59 units operating by the end of 1988, the ARA Corporation would have 61 by the end of 1989, and Manor Care planned to have 13 units by the end of 1988. This would make a total of 133 dementia units in the major for-profit nursing home chains. The author went on to say that the American Association of Homes for the Aging (AAHA) had identified 18 of its nonprofit member nursing homes with units, making a grand total of at least 151 dementia units nationwide. On the other hand, Leon et al. (1990) estimated that 7.6 percent of homes nationally had specialized units and that as many as 14 percent will have such units by 1991.

Our study planned to use a five-state sample to estimate the number of dementia units nationwide. The results would be helpful for those involved in developing policy and for purposes of new research in the field.

2. *To determine the range of variability of current dementia units in terms of auspices, size, age of program, unit goals, admission policies, physical/ environmental properties or modifications, staffing, routine treatment programs, range of service, and costs; to determine the mean, median, and frequency distribution, when applicable, for the above characteristics; to determine the extent that existing dementia units differ from traditional nursing home units.*

Before beginning the project, we spoke to several persons managing dementia units and heavily involved in their development. Our preliminary findings indicated great diversity in what providers of care listed as components of a good program. There was controversy in basic questions such as staffing ratios and the expected outcomes of care provided.

Our study attempted to describe this variability and to provide more precise data on the day-to-day operation of dementia units in the five states sampled. By contrasting the dementia units with settings providing traditional care, we also hoped to identify differences. Documenting the activity of the units would assist in the eventual establishment of minimum standards of care for demented nursing home residents.

3. *To determine the characteristics of dementia unit program participants in terms of demographics, functional status, activity level, mobility status, diagnoses, behavioral problems, and physical and chemical restraint use; to determine how these compare with characteristics of nursing home residents in traditional settings.*

In an attempt to measure the effectiveness of the units, several resident care outcomes were delineated. Although controversy existed over the expectations of care, there were several reasons to measure differences in the nursing home resident populations. Most experts we spoke with testified to the benefits of dementia units, at least in terms of a decrease in problem behaviors and in restraint use. These units, however, can be more costly than traditional care. The results of comparisons between specialized and traditional care would be helpful to administrators trying to decide on the potential benefits of a unit. Our study hoped to describe the differences and to begin to establish whether the dementia unit environment provided an improved approach to problems often faced in the care of Alzheimer's victims.

4. *To determine from 30 dementia unit site visits, and from consultation with experts in the care of demented nursing home residents, what structural and process variables are thought to characterize successful units.*

Our study was designed to provide data on the abilities of dementia unit participants as well as those in traditional settings. By examining these data and through the use of consultants, we hoped to establish which elements of the dementia unit environment were associated with better resident care outcomes.

5. *Based on the information learned from this survey, to identify strategies and measures that can be used to study the effectiveness of dementia units.*

Sampling

Five states were chosen for inclusion in the study: California, New York, North Carolina, Ohio, and Texas. These represented different geographic areas, yet each was among the 10 most populous U.S. states. Use of multiple states would provide a good representation in resident demographics, Medicaid and Medicare reimbursement patterns, and other trends that often are dictated by the regions in which nursing homes are located.

We found that there was no directory of dementia units from which we could draw a sample. Consequently, our first task was to create a list of current nursing homes operating a unit for dementia residents.

For each state, a current directory of all nursing homes was obtained from the licensing office. Telephone calls were then made to every nursing home in each of the five states. Approximately 1400 nursing homes were called in California, 850 in New York, 220 in North Carolina, 1000 in Ohio, and 1022 in Texas. When nursing homes acknowledged having a dementia unit, they were asked a set of questions designed to describe further qualities that are often characteristic of such units.

CRITERIA FOR INCLUSION

Through consultation with professionals who had designed and operated dementia units, specific criteria for inclusion were established. Nursing homes meeting these criteria were included on our final list of dementia units eligible for participation in the project. The criteria involved the following:

1. *The nursing home must identify itself as having a dementia unit.* During the telephone survey, we identified possible dementia units by first asking whether the home had a special area or program for residents with Alzheimer's disease or other dementing illnesses. Terms such as "Alzheimer's Unit," or "Special Care Unit," were often used by such pro-

grams but were not required to meet this criterion. If an entire home was dedicated primarily to dementia treatment, it too was included on our list.

2. *The program must contain a majority of residents with a dementia diagnosis.* Nursing homes were asked what percentage of residents in the unit had some type of dementia. For a variety of reasons, some "dementia units" include residents with disorders other than dementia, such as schizophrenia, stroke, or manic-depressive illness. We believed that in any dementia unit we studied a majority of participants should be diagnosed with a dementing illness. Therefore, to meet this criterion, the unit must have had at least 51 percent of participants with dementia.

3. *The unit should be physically separated from other resident care areas.* Nursing homes were asked if the unit was separated from the rest of the facility either by closed doors or an alarm system, and whether the physical structure was different in any way from the rest of the facility. We believed that a separate living and sleeping area was required to meet the definition of a dementia unit. Thus, we did not study homes with day programs for dementia residents.

4. *The unit should employ a majority of nursing staff with training or experience in geriatric care.* Nursing homes were asked what percentage of the dementia unit staff had more than one year of experience working with geriatric residents. To meet this criterion, homes must have had at least 51 percent of staff having more than one year of experience. This question gave us an indication of the background of workers chosen for the unit. The heavy demands often placed on dementia unit staff meant that it was not a place for new or inexperienced workers. The majority of nursing homes we spoke with met this criterion. However, the high turnover rate for nursing staff in long-term care facilities as a whole caused many study units to have ongoing staff recruitment and training needs.

5. *Unit personnel should receive training in dementia care.* Nursing homes were also asked whether the unit's staff received training in how to care for dementia residents before they began to work on the unit. This criterion was also set at 51 percent. While the majority answered in the affirmative, the training varied greatly in terms of actual hours spent in either didactic or clinical settings.

6. *Unit activities should be designed with the dementia resident in mind.* Nursing homes were asked to what extent the activities on the unit were specifically designed for dementia residents. Possible responses were: all, most, some, or none of the activities. From consultation with experts in the field, we concluded that the daily unit routines such as meals, activities, and rest times should acknowledge the need for flexibility, consistency, and careful planning to preserve remaining function of the

demented residents. If units had all, most, or some of the activities planned specifically for dementia residents, they met this criterion.

Since we wanted to describe the range of existing programs, we allowed some flexibility in our inclusion criteria. Thus, we decided that to be eligible for the study, nursing homes must meet the first two criteria. If they also met three out of the remaining four criteria, they could be included.

New units take some time to develop programs and to admit residents. For this reason, we did not want to visit newly opened dementia units. Therefore, we included an additional criterion related to the length of time a dementia unit had been operational. Specifically, *the dementia unit must have been opened at least six months before our visit.* To determine this, all nursing homes that acknowledged having a unit were asked in what month and year the unit began operating. We believed that a unit would take a minimum of six months to get established and did not want common problems that often affect a new service to interfere with study results. The first six months of operation represented a stage of new growth and change; it was not a time in which to be evaluated. Staff members selected and trained for the unit require time to adjust to their roles and to begin functioning as a team. Assessment forms, procedures to follow, and even changes in the physical structure may require time before their actual value can be determined. Consequently, if a dementia unit met the other criteria but not this one, it was included in the census of all dementia units identified in the state but excluded from the final list of those eligible for a site visit.

The study also intended to compare nonprofit dementia units with those in for-profit (proprietary) homes. For this reason, our telephone screening obtained information on ownership. Nursing homes were asked if they were nonprofit (such as government or church-related facilities), or for profit (such as those owned by an individual or a corporation). The final list of facilities with dementia units in a state was subdivided into for-profit and nonprofit categories.

Government facilities such as Veterans Administration (VA) nursing homes and state, city, or county nursing homes with units were excluded from a visit. The majority of such homes are operated by the VA. These facilities operate in a reimbursement and regulatory environment that is quite different from that of most nursing homes. Therefore, they would be difficult to compare with other nursing homes in our sample. Thus government sponsorship became the final criterion by which nursing homes were excluded from our study sample.

Out of 151 total dementia units identified in all five states, only 11 units did not meet the inclusion criteria. In California, three units in the for-profit sector did not have a majority of participants with a dementia

TABLE A.1   Dementia Units Identified in Each State

	California	New York	North Carolina	Ohio	Texas	Total
Nursing homes in state	1,400	850	220	1,000	1,022	4,492
No. dementia units identified	35	17	8	46	45	151
For-profit	27	4	5	24	32	92
Nonprofit	8	13	3	22	13	59
Units meeting inclusion criteria	32	15	7	41	45	140
For-profit	24	4	5	23	32	88
Nonprofit	8	11	2	18	13	52
Units excluded from study	3	2	1	5	0	11
For-profit	3	0	0	1	0	4
Nonprofit	0	2	1	4	0	7

diagnosis. Two nonprofit units in New York and one in North Carolina were excluded because they were government owned. In Ohio, five units were excluded; one for-profit and one nonprofit unit did not have a majority of participants with a dementia diagnosis, and three nonprofit units were less than six months old when our site visits were made. All units in Texas met the inclusion criteria. Table A.1 summarizes the selection data for each of the five states studied.

SELECTING THE SAMPLE OF FACILITIES WITH DEMENTIA UNITS

Nursing homes on the final list of those eligible for the study were each assigned a number. Using a table of random numbers, we then chose three for-profit and three nonprofit nursing homes from each state for participation in the study. We also chose two alternate homes in each category, in case one or more of the chosen homes refused to participate. Thus, the units in the study represented a stratified random sample of nongovernment dementia units in the five study states.

Administrators of the nursing homes chosen were then contacted by telephone. If they expressed willingness to participate or wanted further details, a packet of written information was sent to them. This packet included a letter explaining the study and the process of a typical half-day site visit. It also included data collection instruments to be used by the nursing home staff, should they agree to participate. Administrators received a follow-up call two weeks after the written information was mailed to inquire about questions and to solicit participation. For those nursing homes agreeing to participate, a tentative date and time for the visit was arranged.

SELECTING THE COMPARISON FACILITIES

Because the study was to be comparative, our next task after selecting dementia units was to identify units for a control group. We wanted the control group to represent "usual and customary" nursing home care. Ideally, it should be the type of care the residents in dementia units would receive if they were not in a dementia unit.

Although we were uncertain, we believed that nursing homes with dementia units may differ from the average U.S. nursing home. They might be larger, have more financial resources, be more progressive, or be in a more competitive environment. If so, the homes themselves would represent a treatment factor. We did not want our study to find differences that arose because the nursing homes in our study group were different from those in our control group. For this reason, we employed a rather elaborate matching scheme designed to select homes for our control group that were similar to the homes that contained our dementia units. We called our control group (homes without dementia units) comparison units. Therefore, the study design involved selecting a sample of three nonprofit and three for-profit homes with dementia units in each state, and then matching them with similar nursing homes not having units (i.e., providing traditional care) for their dementia residents.

Once the sample of six dementia units was chosen and administrators gave consent, the process of matching dementia unit nursing homes with comparison nursing homes was begun. Administrators of the nursing homes having dementia units were asked for the facility Medicaid percentage rate. This information, together with ownership status, geographic locality, and total bed capacity, were key descriptors that we felt might affect policies, procedures, and available resources of the nursing homes. Dementia unit homes were matched with comparison unit homes according to the following criteria: (1) Comparison nursing homes should have a similar proportion of Medicaid recipients as the dementia unit homes they were paired with, ideally within 20 percent. (2) The ownership status (for profit or nonprofit) of both homes in a pair should be the same. (3) Both homes had to be within the same city or county. In rural counties having only one or two nursing homes, or where no appropriate match was possible, homes in adjoining counties were sometimes used. (4) Facility size should be similar. Three sizes were established—

small, medium, and large. Small facilities had fewer than 75 beds, medium-size facilities had 75 to 200 beds, and large facilities had more than 200 beds. (5) Since we had not actually seen the facilities, we were concerned that we might match nursing homes that seem unlike in other ways, such as overall decor, age of the building, and type of person likely to choose the facility. We needed an impartial opinion and decided that the local nursing home ombudsmen might be helpful in this regard. The ombudsmen were familiar with the demographic characteristics of the residents of a facility in general and had visited the homes. The opinion of this person became the final item on which nursing homes were matched.

Within each comparison facility, our site visit selected an area for study that we called the comparison unit. This was an area with defined geographic bounds, usually by virtue of being serviced by one nursing station. Often it consisted of a wing, a floor, or one hall. In selecting the comparison unit to study, we looked for a unit that was at the same level of care as its paired dementia unit and that contained, in the nursing director's opinion, many residents with dementia. Thus, unit level of care was a final matching criterion.

In each of the five states, our goal was to choose three nonprofit and three for-profit dementia units, for a total of 30 units. Matching these nursing homes with an equal number would then give us a grand total of 60 homes nationwide. However, in actuality, we visited 31 units and 32 comparison units. One extra dementia unit and two additional comparison units were visited in North Carolina for reasons that will be discussed below.

REFUSALS AND OTHER POSSIBLE SOURCES OF SAMPLING BIAS

In selecting our dementia unit sample, we contacted 37 facilities to obtain our sample of 31. Thus, the refusal rate was 16 percent for the dementia unit sample. In selecting comparison facilities, we approached 41 homes to obtain our sample of 32. Thus, the refusal rate for comparison facilities was 22 percent.

Administrators of the nursing homes with specialized units often seemed pleased that the study was being conducted; they were eager to describe the contribution they felt dementia units were making to the nursing home industry. During telephone conversations made to prepare the site visits, they often shared additional information about the history, operation, and unique features of their unit.

For obvious reasons, administrators of potential comparison units did not always show similar interest. Some, however, seemed familiar with the concept of dementia units and wanted to gain a better understanding of their value in resident care. A few administrators of comparison homes agreed to participate purely for altruistic reasons.

During the process of matching the dementia units with comparison units, problems emerged with matching on all criteria. For unknown reasons, nursing homes with dementia units seemed to have a larger than average bed capacity. Because our study attempted to match homes in terms of size, the number of homes available to serve as potential comparisons was limited. In both California and New York, two of the six dementia units selected were not matched according to size. One of the six homes selected in Ohio was not matched in regard to size. In North Carolina, two out of seven dementia units were not matched in regard to size. Four homes in Texas were not matched in regard to size.

The Medicaid percentage for the entire facility also seemed to differ for homes with dementia units. Each state showed a consistent trend for homes with dementia units to contain lower proportions of Medicaid residents. The criterion for matching homes by Medicaid proportion was for the comparison home to be within 20 percent of the dementia unit home. This was not possible in three out of six homes in California and Texas, and in three homes out of seven in North Carolina. In New York, only one mismatch (out of six homes) occurred, and none occurred in Ohio.

Occasionally, we had a problem finding a match in the same city or county. Finding suitable comparison homes meant traveling to adjoining counties once in New York, four times in North Carolina, three times in Ohio, once in Texas, and not at all in California. This usually happened when a home chosen for inclusion was in a rural location where fewer nursing homes were available from which comparison homes could be selected.

Some states, such as California and Texas, have more for-profit than nonprofit nursing homes, limiting the available matches for a dementia unit in a nonprofit home. As a result, additional travel time was required to reach an appropriate match with regard to ownership.

In summary, the following mismatches occurred. Among our 31 nursing home pairs, there were no mismatches by state, 2 mismatches by certification level, 3 mismatches by ownership, 10 mismatches by facility size, and 12 mismatches by Medicaid proportion.

Contacting the local nursing home ombudsmen proved extremely helpful. For the most part, these workers were knowledgeable about the homes we had selected, seemed interested in the study, and assisted greatly in finding appropriate comparison homes. In each state, the best matches were found when the ombudsman was active in the selection. Consequently, when matching criteria were not met, the ombudsman's recommendations were followed.

TABLE A.2   Similarity of Comparison Unit Subjects to Senile Dementia or Chronic Organic Brain Syndrome Residents from the 1985 National Nursing Home Survey

Characteristic	Comparison Unit Residents ($N = 318$)	Nursing Home Residents with Dementia ($N - 2302$)
Mean age (yr)	83.2	83.0
Mean length of stay this admission (days)	832	1034
Female (%)	82.1	76.0
Married with living spouse (%)	15.3	14.5
Race (%)		
White	86.8	89.9
Black	8.8	7.1
Other	4.4	4.0
Needing help with (%)		
Dressing	92.5	89.0
Getting out of bed	77.5	71.2
Ambulation	60.4	54.5
Toileting	83.6	71.0
Impaired recent memory by nurse report (%)	87.5	75.8
Current problem with physically abusive behavior (%)	16.4	17.6
Medicaid primary payer (%)	65.7	54.1

NONRANDOM SELECTION OF COMPARISON SITES

Although the dementia unit nursing homes in the study were selected at random, the homes without dementia units were not. Thus our set of comparison homes cannot be used to estimate the status of nursing home care in our study states. Instead, the data collected describe a group of demented residents who are receiving usual and customary care in homes similar to the homes that have dementia units.

On the other hand, our comparison unit residents appear to be very much like typical dementia residents in nursing homes nationwide. When our comparison group subjects were compared with national estimates for all nursing home residents with "senile dementia or chronic organic brain syndrome" from the 1985 National Nursing Home Survey, the two populations were remarkably similar. Table A.2 summarizes a variety of key demographic and functional status variables for these two groups. Differences are relatively minor, particularly in functional status, cognitive status, and the prevalence of behavioral problems, which are key determinants of care requirements. Thus, while population estimates cannot be made from our comparison group data, the residents in our comparison group are likely to be representative of the overall population of dementia residents in U.S. nursing homes.

A more ideal study design would have been to have two comparison groups, one consisting of units in the same homes as the dementia units but not providing specialized dementia care, and the other a random sample of all long-term care facilities in the study state. This work is being planned for the future. The present study, however, was designed to be descriptive as much as comparative. Consequently, we sought to obtain the most appropriate single comparison group possible in order to spend more effort learning abut the specialized units themselves.

Measures to Protect Resident Rights and Assure Confidentiality

Protection of rights and prevention of injury are particularly important in research on people with dementing illness. When such research poses any risk to subjects, informed consent should be obtained. Our study was reviewed twice during its planning stages by the Committee for the Protection of the Rights of Human Subjects of the University of North Carolina School of Medicine (UNC). The study was specifically designed not to require any interaction with study subjects or to provide any changes in care. Furthermore, all data collected were identified by number rather than name so that confidentiality could be preserved. Because of the nonintrusive nature and confidentiality safeguards of our study, the UNC Human Subjects Committee believed that individual consent of subjects was not required.

Nevertheless, a few facilities wanted to obtain permission from family members, largely because they believed we should have permission before entering medical records of the residents. The National Nursing Home Survey avoids this issue by requiring staff to search records for responses to interviewers' questions, but we did not want to place such a time burden on facilities and performed our own medical record reviews. Thus, in some facilities our study sample was drawn randomly in advance and families were approached for permission, usually by telephone. In all such cases the facility administrators were helpful in obtaining permission.

Site Visits

Most of the study data were collected during a half-day site visit. Each visit was conducted by either Dr. Philip Sloane (33 visits), Laura

Mathew (25 visits), or Eunice Grossman (7 visits). To standardize data collection and reduce inter-rater error, two pilot site visits (data not reported here) and two of the data collection site visits were made together by pairs of co-investigators.

We attempted to standardize site visits as much as possible. The visits all occurred during the work week (Monday through Friday). Because of the unusual amount of volunteer activity before Christmas, no site visits were conducted between the first week of December and the 4th of January. Half of both the dementia units and comparison units were visited in the morning, and half in the afternoon. In all cases, the same investigator collected data on both members of a dementia unit–comparison unit pair.

A typical site visit lasted three or four hours. It began with the investigator meeting with the facility administrator to review the goals of the study and discuss the activities that would take place during the site visit. If a specific unit had not been chosen beforehand for the site visit, as was true in many of the comparison homes, a unit was identified. Next, the site visitor was introduced to a staff member who would provide assistance in the data collection. That staff member, usually a nurse, assisted in constructing the study sample, oriented the investigator to the unit, helped identify subjects for nonparticipant observation, and assisted with the completion of the Multidimensional Observation Scale for Elderly Subjects (Helmes et al. 1987), which is discussed in the following section on instruments.

Next, a census of residents with dementing illness was constructed for the unit. A dementia diagnosis was determined to be present if one of the following terms or an abbreviation of it was listed on the admission or face sheet, history and physical, hospital discharge summary, or nursing care plan: Alzheimer's disease, multi-infarct dementia, senile dementia, senility, dementia, organic brain syndrome, chronic brain syndrome, primary degenerative dementia, chronic confusion, or cerebral arteriosclerosis.

From the list of residents with dementia, ten study subjects were chosen using a table of random numbers. (In a few cases, data were collected on only eight or nine subjects because of unit size or informed consent issues.) On each of these study subjects, a medical record review form, a nonparticipant observation form, and the Multidimensional Observation Scale for Elderly Subjects (MOSES) were completed during the site visit. In addition, five dementia residents randomly chosen from a list of the 10 most recent discharges from the study unit were identified, and with the assistance of the facility medical records clerk, certain data on each were obtained. (In a number of facilities visited, we obtained data on fewer than five recent discharges because the unit was relatively new or the records were difficult to identify and retrieve.)

Sometime during each site visit, two observational periods occurred. During one observational period the investigator, guided by a staff member, observed the ten subjects in as unobtrusive a manner as possible and completed a nonparticipant observation form for each subject. During the other observational period, the investigator walked about the unit collecting data on the physical environment and on staff and resident activities. The nonparticipant observation forms are discussed further in the following section on instruments.

The typical visit concluded with a visit to the administrator, during which the administrative questionnaire was reviewed. Each facility received a small reimbursement to help defray personnel costs incurred in the data collection process.

During our site visits, we were impressed with the professionalism, cordiality, and openness of virtually all the many administrators and staff with whom we worked. Both dementia unit facilities and those in the comparison group were extremely helpful, often in spite of many competing time demands. Thanks in large measure to the help of these dedicated and concerned professionals, we were successful in carrying out the rather ambitious data collection requirements of our site visits.

Instruments and Data Collection

Eight separate instruments were used in the study: a telephone survey form, an administrative questionnaire for homes with dementia units, an administrative questionnaire for homes without dementia units, a medical record review form for current residents, a medical record review form for discharged residents, a resident observation form, the MOSES scale, and a unit observation form. Each is described below. The procedure followed as data were collected for each form is also discussed.

TELEPHONE SURVEY

A telephone survey was used to identify dementia units in each state. Every nursing home in the five states was asked if a unit was in operation. When homes responded affirmatively, an administrative staff member or the social worker was asked about the program.

In addition to routine identifying information, such as name and address, the homes were asked about their ownership in terms of for-profit and nonprofit status and the month and year the unit was opened. They were then asked to estimate the percentage of residents in the unit with some type of dementing illness. Questions about the staff working on the unit included the estimated percentage of staff with more than one year of experience in geriatric patient care and the percentage of staff who received training in dementia care before they began working on the unit. Questions pertaining to structure included whether or not the unit was separated by closed doors, an alarm system, or other means from the rest of the home and whether or not any changes had been made in the physical layout (such as walls, carpeting, or other design elements) exclusively for the unit. Finally, homes were asked to estimate what percentage of activities were designed specifically for demented residents.

Our sampling frame of for-profit and nonprofit homes meeting the criteria for inclusion was derived from this data. The identifying information was used to contact administrators of homes chosen and request permission to visit. Preliminary information gathered with this form was then verified with administrators.

Data were collected on the telephone survey form by a group of student research assistants and other project staff. Students assisting with the project were trained by the project staff. A standardized interview form for questioning the homes was followed. Because of the volume of telephone calls to be made, data collection lasted several months. Additional calls had to be made shortly before contacting administrators and planning the site visits to ensure that the information collected was current. The telephone surveys were completed between December 1987 and August 1988; the site visits were completed between November 1987 and April 1989.

ADMINISTRATIVE QUESTIONNAIRES

Two questionnaires were designed for gathering information from administrators of the homes in the study. Each began with a background section that obtained identifying information and descriptors of the facility, such as bed size, occupancy rates, and certification. A financial section asked about daily charges and reimbursement issues. A staffing section pertained to the number and categories of workers on the nursing home unit to be visited. A section on the physical layout of the facility included the number and types of rooms on the unit and square footage for each. A policies section sought information about the home's involvement with community, research, and educational activities. A section on admissions and discharges obtained estimates of the number and status of residents moved in and out of the unit. Finally, a section on procedures asked the homes to check off which activities were offered from a list including such items as reminiscence therapy and exercise programs.

The administrative questionnaire for homes with dementia units was identical to the one for comparison homes with the exception of six supplemental open-ended questions. These six questions asked administrators or unit directors why the unit was started, what they believed made an ideal unit, what they perceived as the greatest rewards and drawbacks of the unit, what rewards were given to the staff, and what strategies, if any, they used to advertise their unit.

Administrators of the homes selected were first approached by telephone for their permission to visit. If the administrator showed interest in receiving additional information, a letter followed. The administrative questionnaire was sent at this time, and the administrator was asked to complete the form before the site visit. During the site visit, that form was reviewed with the administrator and any questions were answered. On occasion, the form was mailed back to the researchers after the site visit. One facility of the 63 visited did not return its questionnaire.

REVIEW OF CURRENT RESIDENTS' MEDICAL RECORDS

Ten residents currently on the unit were selected at random from a list of all residents having a diagnosis of dementia. The medical records of these ten residents were reviewed by project staff making the site visit. Information gathered included the following: the age, sex, race, and marital status of the resident; the date first admitted to a nursing home; the date of the latest admission; the location of the resident before admission; the diagnoses (up to a total of six); all routinely administered (not PRN) medications, with dosages for psychotropics; the total number medications; the number of hospitalizations and emergency room visits within the past six months as a result of injury or acute illness; the current payment source; the frequency of family visits; and the resident's weight at the time of the visit and three months earlier.

An additional item was the Resource Utilization Groups (RUGs) score, which was calculated for each resident with the assistance of a staff member knowledgeable about the resident's abilities. The RUGs system was devised by Fries and Cooney (1985) and is used in some states for reimbursement. The RUGs score estimates the amount of time nursing staff spend with a resident by placing the resident in one of sixteen care categories.

In addition to the RUGs score, a number of other items on the medical record review form had to be obtained or verified for accuracy by asking the nursing staff. These items included hospitalization rates, the current marital status, and the frequency of family visits. Nursing staff were asked to rate the frequency of family visits on a four-point scale, beginning at "daily visits" and ending at "once a month or less." Personnel in the administrative office were asked to verify the current payment source of the resident. At times the social worker was asked about the resident's background, such as where the resident was before admission, if this was not found in the record. The medical records staff was also consulted when the record had been thinned and notes reflected only one or two months of activity.

REVIEW OF PAST RESIDENTS' MEDICAL RECORDS

To describe the population of residents who were moved off both the dementia and comparison units, the records of former residents were also reviewed. The records of residents with a dementia diagnosis from both settings were reviewed. Five records were chosen at random from a list of the 10 most recent discharges. Less information was gathered on this group than on current residents. Data collected for past residents included the age at discharge, sex, race, where the resident was taken at the time of discharge, the reason for discharge, and the length of stay for that admission. Data on this form were collected by project staff; because previous records were consulted, assistance was required from the home's medical records worker.

THE MOSES SCALE

The Multidimensional Observation Scale for Elderly Subjects (MOSES) developed by Helmes et al. (1987) was used to gather information on the ten current residents chosen at random for medical record review. The MOSES scale has five dimensions on which the resident's abilities are rated. These five dimensions are activities of daily living, cognitive ability, emotional and behavioral status, and interactions with others. When tested by Helmes et al. (1987) among 2,542 people, the MOSES was found to be an objective, valid, and reliable instrument that could be used for assessment, placement, monitoring, and research. Most of the 40 questions in the MOSES have four possible responses; a few have a fifth possible response, usually one indicating that none of the others are applicable. The resident's abilities are rated on the basis of these responses. For example, the first item, which relates to dressing, states: "On most days in the past week, the resident (1) initiated and completed dressing without supervision, (2) dressed with only minor supervision, (3) partly dressed himself, but needed frequent staff assistance, or (4) was either totally dressed by staff or remained in bedclothes."

The MOSES must be completed by someone knowledgeable about the resident's abilities. For this reason, nursing staff on the units were asked to gather these data. This was done during the site visit. Approximately 10 minutes was spent per resident in completing the MOSES scales. Project staff provided instruction and reviewed data for accuracy and completeness.

NONPARTICIPANT RESIDENT OBSERVATION

A nonparticipant resident observation form was used to describe the appearance of the same 10 residents chosen at random for record review and for completion of the MOSES scale. Because the project staff did not know the 10 residents, a nursing staff member was asked to point them out. Residents were not interviewed, and observation was as unobtrusive as possible. Initially, behavior was observed from as far away as possible. Then the investigator moved closer to observe grooming and restraint status.

The project staff (investigator) making the visit noted the location of the resident on a checklist. The activity of the resident was also recorded in terms of whether or not any interaction, passive or active, was taking place, and whether interaction was with another resident, a staff member, or a visitor. The resident's mobility status (in bed, walking, in a wheelchair, in a geri-chair, in another chair) was noted. In addition, whether the resident was physically restrained at the time of the observation was noted. The resident's personal grooming was evaluated in three areas: overall cleanliness, hair, and clothing; each was rated on a three point scale. The resident's level of awareness was noted, and observed behavioral characteristics were recorded on a checklist of possible symptoms including wandering, moaning, talking to self, aggressiveness, quarrelsomeness, and pacing. Other observed symptoms could be written in.

The collection of observation data lasted about one minute per resident. Data were collected at a consistent time during each site visit avoiding meal times and shift changes. The morning observations were done at about 10:00 or 10:30. The afternoon observations were done either at about 2:00 or after 3:30, avoiding the routine activities associated with shift change.

THE UNIT OBSERVATION QUESTIONNAIRE

The unit observation questionnaire described activity on the unit as a whole and the physical environment. All residents, as opposed to only the 10 chosen at random, and all staff members present, were noted. This scale had two sections; one focused on the people of the unit, and the other on the environment.

The first section described the activities of residents and staff. Residents could be either in public areas or in their own rooms. Those in public areas such as dayrooms, hallways, or dining rooms were noted to be in one of the following situations: sitting, not participating; sitting, actively participating; standing or walking alone; standing or walking with others; or in some other situation that could be written in and described. For residents in private areas such as their own rooms, the following situations were possible: in bed, interacting with a roommate or visitor; in bed, with staff attending; in bed, alone; out of bed, interacting with a roommate or visitor; out of bed, with staff; out of bed, alone or not interacting; in the bathroom, alone; or in the bathroom, with staff attending. The privacy of the residents was honored; closed doors to residents' rooms were not opened. Thus, only those residents in rooms with open doors were studied. The total number of residents observed was recorded, as was the unit census. This gave us an estimate of the percentage of residents on the unit we had observed.

The number of staff and volunteers on the unit at the time of the observation was also documented. As with the residents, the activity level of the staff and volunteers was described; they were either interacting directly with residents or involved in other activities. The number of total staff and volunteers observed was recorded. Sitters hired by families were not included as staff. This number gave us an estimate of the staff–resident ratio at the time of the observation.

Environmental elements included in the unit observation were: lighting, noise, odor, glare on floors, amount of personal items in resident rooms, and amount of homelike furnishings on the unit. These items were rated on a three-point scale. In addition, other physical attributes of the unit were: whether or not the unit was separated by closed doors, had a courtyard or access to the outdoors, had a wandering path, had small group discussion areas, had a television on, or had a kitchen available for residents' use.

An additional item requested information from the charge nurse of the unit. The nurse was asked to give an estimate of the number of residents on the unit who were presently being treated for stage two pressure sores or other areas of skin breakdown.

The unit observation was conducted by the project staff member making the site visit. This task lasted about 15 minutes. The investigator walked up and down hallways and through all public areas to collect information. The unit observation was conducted at about the same time as the resident observations, avoiding meal times and shift changes.

SUBJECTIVE NOTES

In addition to the objective measurements discussed above, additional information was collected in the form of personal and subjective notes describing each site visit. These notes, written by the project staff member, described impressions of the nursing home and the unit visited. They often focused on individual strengths or weaknesses that were perceived, remarked on the nuances of the unit, posed questions about the research itself, provided additional descriptions, or gave examples. In each case, the subjective notes supplemented the more objective data already collected with the various instruments. These notes were compiled immediately after the visit while the impressions were easily remembered.

Data collected in subjective notes were helpful in organizing descriptions of all nursing homes in the study. Together with the more objective findings, these data helped us develop the typology of nursing homes discussed in chapter 3.

NATIONAL COMPARISON DATA

To compare our study population with national statistics for nursing home residents, we analyzed data from the 1985 National Nursing Home Survey (NNHS). Residents in the NNHS sample were identified as having dementia if their diagnoses included "senile dementia/chronic and organic brain syndrome." Analyzing this subset of the NNHS, we computed estimates of selected demographic and functional status measures for all dementia residents in U.S. nursing homes.

Data Preparation and Entry

The data collected for each of the eight questionnaires was reviewed by one of the principal investigators and then entered into the computer by means of a database management program. A separate data set was created for each questionnaire, and a number of checks were built into the program to minimize data entry errors. From here on, the data were uploaded to the mainframe computer at the University of North Carolina in Chapel Hill. Statistical Analysis System (SAS) files were created for each questionnaire, and additional checks ascertained the accuracy of information in each data set.

Each of the eight questionnaires contains a clear coding scheme, but in some cases additional codes were created to accommodate valid entries. This was especially true with the medical record review questionnaire, where information was collected on the residents' diagnoses and medications. Codes were developed for diagnoses and medications.

The Project Staff and Consultants

The project staff consisted of six members. Philip D. Sloane, M.D., M.P.H., was the principal investigator. Dr. Sloane is an associate professor in the Departments of Family Medicine and Epidemiology at the University of North Carolina (UNC). Laura J. Mathew, R.N., M.P.H., served as co-investigator and project coordinator. At the time of the study she was a clinical instructor in the Department of Family Medicine, UNC.

Her background is in gerontological and nursing. She is now with UNC Hospitals.

In addition, Eunice Grossman, M.Ed., served as a research associate for the project. At the time of data collection, she was a member of the staff of the Department of Family Medicine at UNC and was coordinating the activities of the Geriatric Education Center of the medical school.

Three project members were from the School of Public Health at UNC. William G. Weissert, Ph.D., provided input on the finances of the long-term care industry, an area in which he has published extensively and is well known. Dr. Weissert is now a professor in the Department of Health Services Management and Policy and a research scientist with the Institute of Gerontology at the University of Michigan in Ann Arbor.

Jaikishan R. Desai, M.P.H., and Margaret Scarborough, M.P.H., served as research assistants for the project and provided data analysis. Both are doctoral students at the UNC School of Public Health and have backgrounds in statistical analysis.

The project was also assisted by a number of consultants who provided valuable guidance. These were: Lisa P. Gwyther, A.C.S.W., and Deborah T. Gold, Ph.D., from Duke University Center for Study on Aging; Carol Hogue, Ph.D., from UNC School of Nursing; Nancy K. Orr, M.S.G., from the Hillhaven Corporation; Nancy Mace, M.A., dementia care consultant in practice; Lorraine G. Hiatt, Ph.D., environmental consultant in practice; and Deborah Beitler, M.A., from the American Association of Homes for the Aging.

References

Fries, B.E., and Cooney, L.M. 1985. Resource Utilization Groups. A patient classification system for long-term care. *Medical Care,* 23: 110–22.

Helmes, E., Csapo, K.G., and Short, J.A. 1987. Standardization and validation of the Multidimensional Observation Scale for Elderly Subjects. *Journal of Gerontology* 42: 395–405.

Leon, J., Potter, D.E.B., and Cunningham, P.J. 1990. *Current and Projected Availability of Special Nursing Home Programs for Alzheimer's Disease Patients.* DHHS publication no. (PHS) 90-3463. National Medical Expenditure Survey Data Summary 1, Agency for Health Care Policy and Research. Rockville, Md: Public Health Service.

U.S. Congress, Office of Technology Assessment. 1987. *Losing a Million Minds: Confronting the Tragedy of Alzheimer's Disease and Other Dementias.* OTA-BA-323. Washington, DC: Government Printing Office.

Wagner, Lynn. 1987. Nursing homes develop special Alzheimer's units. *Modern Healthcare,* April 24: 40–46.

Index